BODY WEIGHT WORKOUTS FOR MEN

SEAN BARTRAM

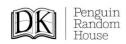

British Edition
Project Editor Kathryn Meeker
Senior Art Editor Glenda Fisher
Angliciser Constance Novis
Senior Pre-production Producer Tony Phipps
Senior Producer Stephanie McConnell
Managing Art Editor Christine Keilty
Managing Editor Stephanie Farrow

American Edition
Publisher Mike Sanders
Associate Publisher Billy Fields
Acquisitions Editor Nathalie Mornu
Copy Editor John Etchison
Jacket Designer Harriet Yeomans
Designer XAB Design
Photographer Matt Bowen
Editorial Assistants/Compositors Ayanna Lacey, Brian Massey
Proofreader Laura Caddell
Indexer Celia McCoy

First published in Great Britain in 2016 by
Dorling Kindersley Limited
80 Strand, London WC2R 0RL

Copyright © 2016 Dorling Kindersley Limited
A Penguin Random House Company
2 4 6 8 10 9 7 5 3 1
001 – 289124 – Jan/2016

A CIP catalogue record for this book is available
from the British Library

ISBN: 978-0-2412-4067-0

Note: This publication contains the opinions and ideas of its author(s). It
is intended to provide helpful and informative material on the subject matter
covered. It is sold with the understanding that the author(s) and publisher
are not engaged in rendering professional services in the book. If the reader
requires personal assistance or advice, a competent professional should
be consulted. The author(s) and publisher specifically disclaim any
responsibility for any liability, loss, or risk, personal or otherwise, which is
incurred as a consequence, directly or indirectly, of the use and application
of any of the contents of this book.

Printed and bound in Hong Kong

All images © Dorling Kindersley Limited
For further information see: www.dkimages.com

A WORLD OF IDEAS:
SEE ALL THERE IS TO KNOW
www.dk.com

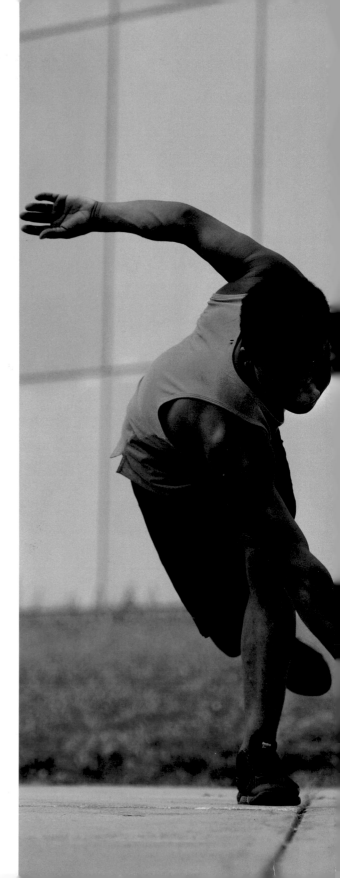

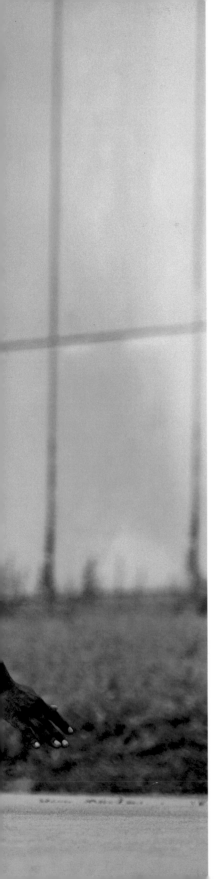

CONTENTS

Level 2   100

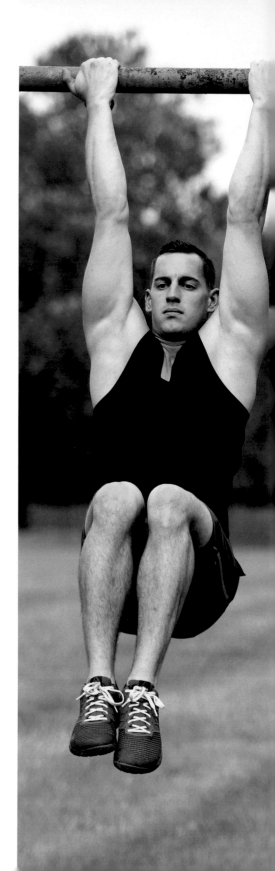

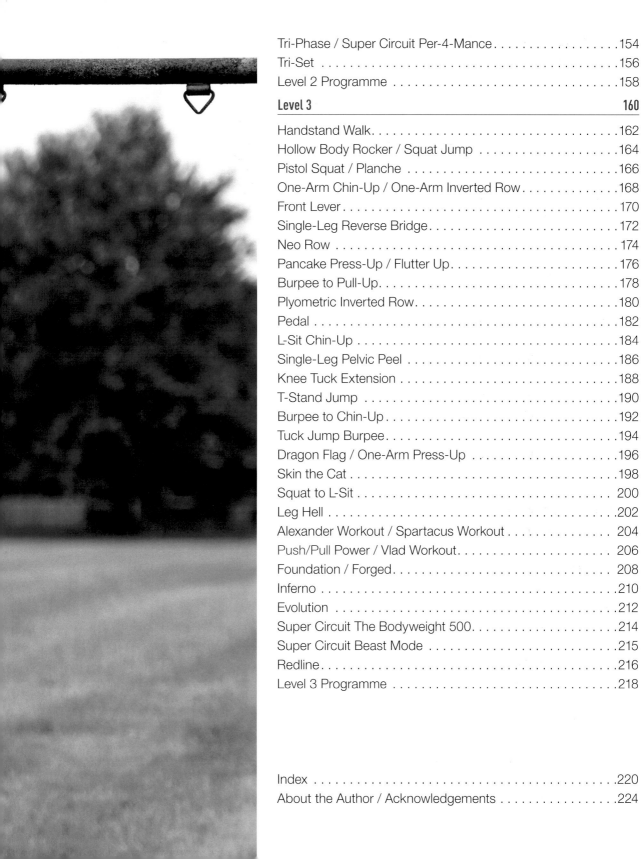

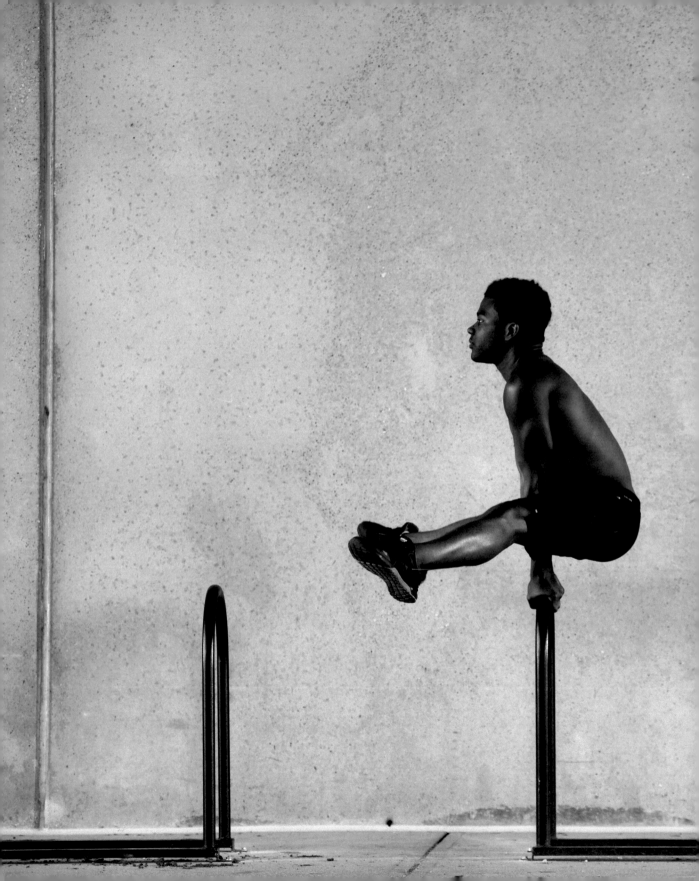

INTRODUCTION

Use the body you've got to get the body you want!

Intimidated by the gym? Short of time or money? Travel frequently? Or just fed up with watching that guy constantly doing bicep curls on the gym's squat rack? Keep reading!

Calisthenics, or bodyweight training, is arguably the world's oldest form of strength training, and now the hottest! Banish the barbells, build lean muscle, decrease body fat, increase performance, and do it all anytime, anywhere.

As a master instructor, I help people from all walks of life to get fit and improve their overall health. My clients include superhuman professional American football players, elite field sport athletes, and professional racing car drivers. They also include men just like you – busy guys who value every second, and to whom efficiency and economy is just as important as body-fat percentage. No matter the goal, I've successfully used the exercises in this book to help my clients reach peak physical fitness!

This book will take you on an incredible journey to a fitter, stronger body using little more than your own bodyweight. Featuring 75 exercises – each with modifications to meet any ability level – 36 unique workouts, and a dynamic 90-day plan, *Bodyweight Workouts for Men* will challenge your perception of strength training and evolve your approach to fitness. I can't promise you it will be easy, but I can promise it will be worth it!

Join the bodyweight revolution!

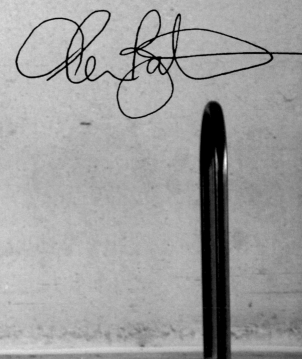

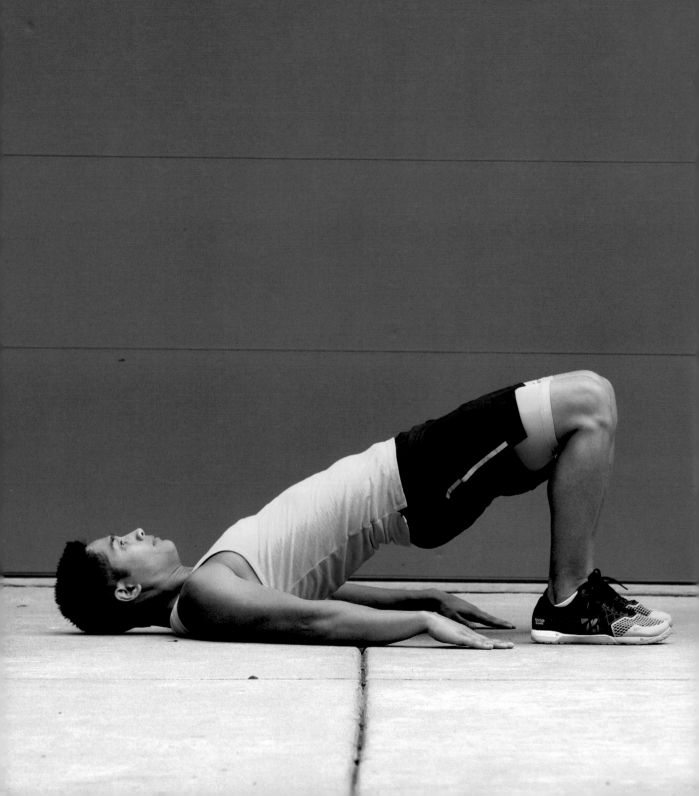

BODYWEIGHT BASICS

The first step in your bodyweight revolution is to understand what you're fighting for. Among other things, this chapter teaches you the "Big Six" exercises, which will form the foundation of your training. It also explains the ways to make any exercise easier or harder with simple, easy-to-follow modifications.

I strongly recommend digesting the information in this chapter, as it will make all your training more effective and efficient.

WHAT IS BODYWEIGHT RESISTANCE TRAINING?

Bodyweight exercises are strength-training exercises that don't require the addition of free weights, such as dumbbells or barbells. The practitioner's own weight provides the resistance for the movements.

Examples of traditional bodyweight resistance exercises include press-ups and pull-ups. The beauty of this training is that for every exercise, there's a simple yet effective way to increase or decrease the exercise's challenge. Take the press-up, for example. To make the exercise less difficult, you can perform a kneeling press-up. To make it more difficult, you have a multitude of options, from changing your hand positions to establishing stops throughout the motion to elevating your feet. These variations not only increase the exercise's difficulty, but also extend the range of motion and recruit more muscle fibres.

In general, increasing the number of repetitions will improve endurance, while strength gains are made by increasing the intensity of the exercise by decreasing leverage, by working at the ends of range of motion, or by adding dynamic tension.

Organizations such as the World Calisthenics Organization and competitions such as Battle of the Bars showcase the elite performance that can be garnered from bodyweight resistance training. Practitioners and legends such as Al Kavadlo, Kenneth Gallarzo, Frank Medrano, and Denis Minin defy gravity on YouTube and other social media sites with physics-bending feats of strength created by utilizing the same techniques presented in this book.

Despite what an entire industry tries to promote, you do not need to pick up a weight to gain strength, increase lean muscle mass, and improve athletic performance.

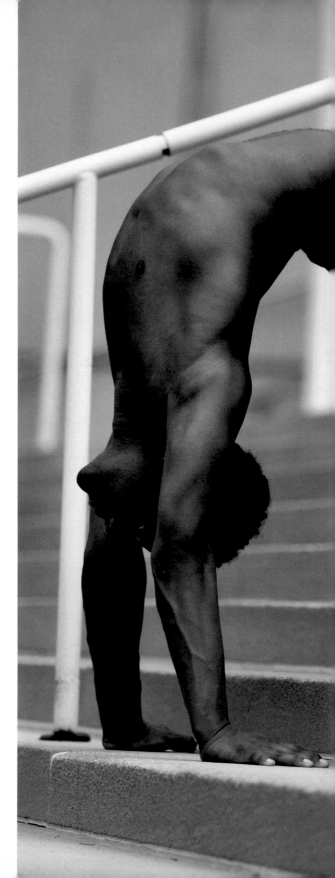

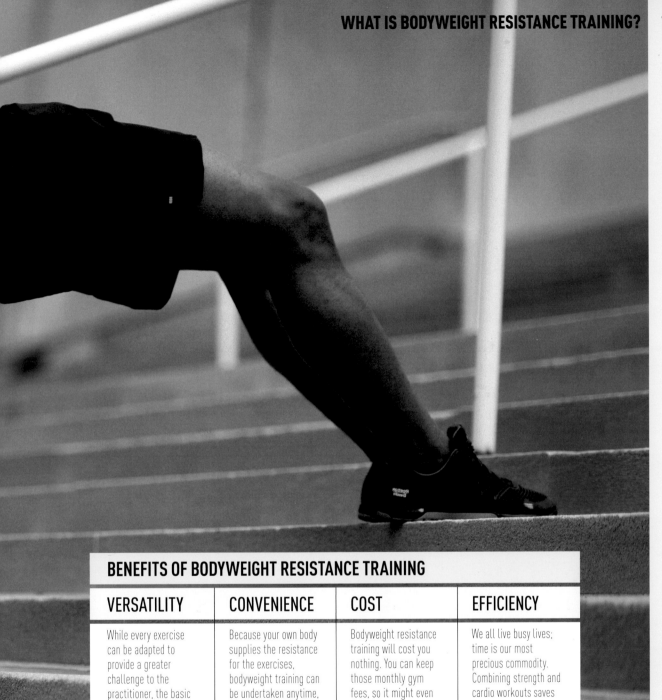

BENEFITS OF BODYWEIGHT RESISTANCE TRAINING

VERSATILITY	CONVENIENCE	COST	EFFICIENCY
While every exercise can be adapted to provide a greater challenge to the practitioner, the basic exercises are also perfect for beginners.	Because your own body supplies the resistance for the exercises, bodyweight training can be undertaken anytime, anywhere – your home, a hotel room, a gym, or in the great outdoors.	Bodyweight resistance training will cost you nothing. You can keep those monthly gym fees, so it might even save you money.	We all live busy lives; time is our most precious commodity. Combining strength and cardio workouts saves time and reduces the transition time between exercises. Most workouts take only 10–45 minutes.

ADVANTAGES OF BODYWEIGHT RESISTANCE TRAINING

Let's be honest. While we work out for the health benefits, a big plus is looking great with your shirt off. Being fit, lean, and healthy boosts self-confidence and makes you want to spend more time training.

I suspect you're interested in decreasing body fat, gaining strength, adding lean muscle, and improving your athletic performance. The exercises and programmes in this book will help you to meet those goals.

ADAPTABILITY

For years the fitness industry portrayed bodyweight exercise as little more than a warm-up, endurance, or cardio workout. The theory was that gaining strength required lifting progressively heavier weights, paying attention to load, not reps. But why can't bodyweight exercises be progressive? Take standard press-ups. Perform as many repetitions as possible in a given time, and it's only about endurance. Increase the time it takes to perform each rep, however, and/or the dynamic tension (the muscular force required to execute that rep), and it makes the exercise more challenging and builds both strength and lean muscle mass, just like adding weight to a barbell. Applying these basic principles to every bodyweight exercise allows you to adapt the resistance and force required.

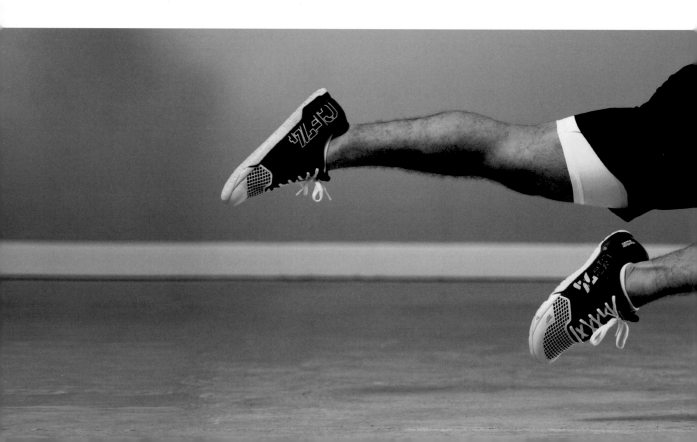

BUILD LEAN MUSCLE AND BURN FAT

You'll work multiple muscle groups at once via compound exercises. The minimal equipment and space required make it easy to transition between exercises, reducing rest time and allowing for a high-intensity interval training type of workout. Alternating sets with minimal or no rest forces the body to produce muscle-building and fat-burning hormones like HGH and testosterone. This also stimulates excess post-exercise oxygen consumption (EPOC, also known as the "afterburn"), the measurable increased rate of oxygen intake following strenuous activity intended to erase the body's oxygen debt. Fatty acids are released as fuel for recovery. EPOC can boost fat burning for up to 48 hours.

INCREASE ATHLETIC PERFORMANCE

Alternating between exercises, working multiple muscle groups per exercise, and the lack of equipment all allow you to keep your body in a state of confusion, preventing it from adapting to a steady workload. Build in easy and simple ways to add or remove challenge and variety through exercise adaptations, and there really are an endless number of ways you can apply the techniques, exercises, and workouts found in this book.

CORE STRENGTH

Consisting of at least 29 muscles, your core is more than just six-pack abs. Every bodyweight exercise featured in this book engages the core either as a primary muscle or for stabilization. This will not only carve the kind of killer core usually seen on models on the front covers of fitness publications, but will also improve your posture and athletic performance.

SYMMETRY

There's no better way to develop a natural, symmetrical, and functional physique. You'll build the lean, athletic, and perfectly proportioned body of a Spartan warrior, gymnast, or martial artist. Research suggests that body symmetry can indicate biological fitness and longer life expectancy – not to mention that studies have shown that humans find symmetrical people more sexually attractive!

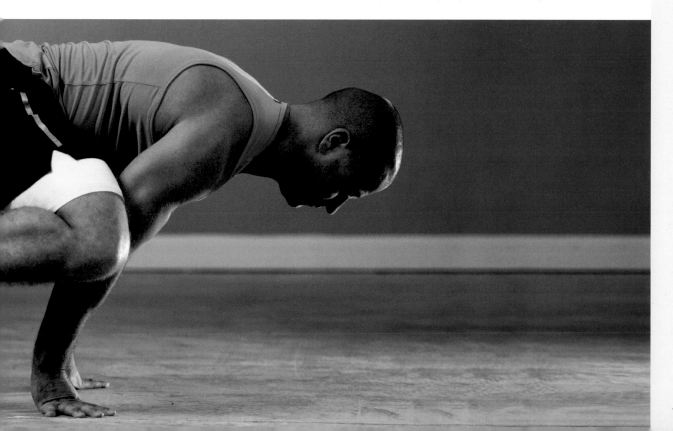

MUST HAVES AND USEFUL EXTRAS

The best part about bodyweight resistance training is that you need little more than your body and a determination to have an incredible workout.

Ingenuity will allow you to use your surroundings, park benches, climbing frames, or chairs to replace the free weights and cardio equipment that keep you mentally and financially chained to your gym membership. However, there are a few optional items I strongly suggest you invest in for optimal performance during the exercises and workouts.

THE MUST HAVES

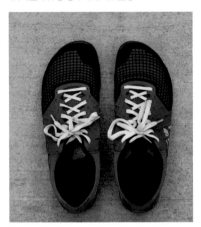

SHOES To make sure you can feel your connection to the floor, I advocate wearing a minimalist-style shoe when training. If you're new to minimalist footwear, I strongly recommend alternating between your old shoes and the minimalist style for two to four weeks to allow your body to adjust to the decrease in support and cushioning.

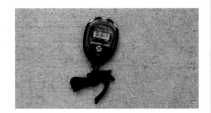

WATCH OR TIMER A watch or timer is essential for keeping track of the work and rest intervals in some workouts.

USEFUL EXTRAS

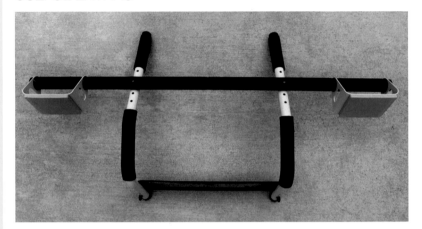

PULL-UP BAR A pull-up bar is not essential, as you can find a number of alternatives for bar-oriented exercises. However, to maximize training performance, I strongly suggest you invest in a door-mounted bar or freestanding pull/dip station.

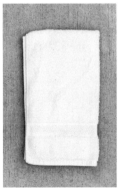

TOWEL In addition to mopping your brow, a towel can also be used to help assist with some exercises.

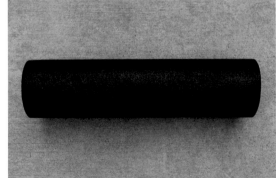

FOAM ROLLER Using a foam roller to provide pre- and/or post-workout myofascial release will increase your performance and decrease your risk of injury.

HOW TO USE THIS BOOK

This book begins with the pertinent questions on the what, when, where, and why of bodyweight resistance training. Please read this information, as it will educate you on the foundation-building "Big Six."

It also explains how to warm up and cool down functionally and how to hydrate and fuel your body correctly. These topics will help you to work out safely, improve your performance, and reduce your recovery time so you can work out more efficiently.

This book presents a plan engineered to take a beginner from Level 1 to Level 3 over a 90-day period, increasing strength, building lean muscle mass, and decreasing body fat along the way.

THE METHOD

1	2	3	4	5
Hydrate and perform functional warm-ups before every workout.	Refer to the first day of the 30-day programme for Level 1 to determine which workout to perform.	Turn to that workout page and perform the exercises it lists, referring as necessary to the individual exercise pages for reference.	After every workout, foam roll for recovery, and hydrate and refuel your body. You're done for today!	Tomorrow, move on to the next day's workout in Level 1. Over the course of a month, complete the exercises in Level 1. Then repeat for Levels 2 and 3.

THE EXERCISES

The exercises are explained with step-by-step photos, and each has a unique more difficult and less difficult version. Review these exercises until they're familiar.

THE WORKOUTS

Workouts vary in length, style, and format to keep your body on its toes. Some have built-in finishers, short metabolic-boosting sets, and core circuits that target your abs but also your back, hips, glutes, and other stabilizing muscles.

THE PROGRAMMES

The three programmes are shown in an easy-to-follow graphical guide for each level. Each one provides a comprehensive 30-day plan. Combined across all levels, they create a 90-day bodyweight evolution.

Q&A

What if I can't perform every exercise or every rep at the end of the 28-day period?
You can either repeat the level and extend your overall commitment, or move on to the next level and continue to substitute any exercise from the previous level until you have it mastered.

What do I do after 90 days?
Start again, but this time perform all the more challenging progressions for each exercise, or create your own workouts.

What should I do on my rest day?
Enjoy it! It has been hard earned. And definitely foam roll and recover.

ANATOMICAL CHART

Throughout these pages, you'll find mentions of the various muscle groups strengthened and developed by bodyweight exercises. The diagrams here will help you understand musculature and general anatomy.

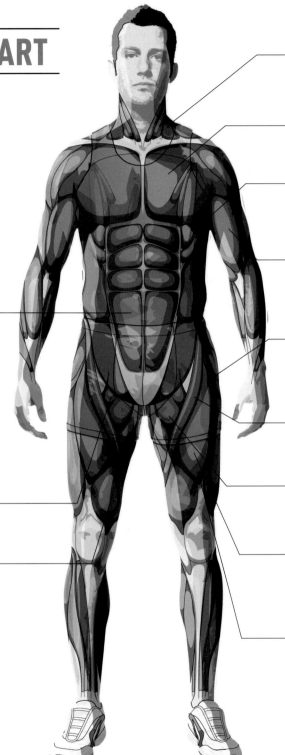

Trapezius

Pectorals – Pectoralis major and pectoralis minor help move the shoulder joint.

Serratus anterior – Originating between the first and ninth ribs, it inserts at the shoulder blade and moves and stabilizes it.

Biceps – This two-headed muscle is responsible for shoulder flexion, elbow flexion, and upwards rotation of the palm.

Tensor fascia latae – This thigh muscle helps stabilize the pelvis atop the femur (thigh bone) while standing.

Sartorius – The longest muscle in the body, it assists in flexion and lateral rotation of the hip, and flexion of the knee.

Pectineus – This flat, quadrangular muscle moves the thigh towards the body and rotates it towards the centre.

Quadriceps – Comprised of the rectus femoris, vastus lateralis, vastus intermedius, and vastus medialis, which extend the knee.

Rectus femoris – See Quadriceps.

The abdominals consist of the following three groups:

Rectus abdominis – Also known as the "six-pack," this runs the length of the front of the abdomen and is important for posture. Its primary function is flexion of the lumbar spine.

Internal and external obliques – Found on the lateral and anterior portions of the abdomen, these pull the chest downwards and compress the abdominal cavity, providing strength and support for the abdomen and spine.

Transversus abdominus – The innermost of the flat muscles of the abdomen compresses the ribs, providing thoracic and pelvic stability.

Illiopsoas (hip flexor) – A combination of the psoas major and illiacus, and essential to athletic activities like running because they're the strongest flexors of the thigh at the hip joint.

Adductors – Commonly called the inner thigh, this group of muscles includes the adductor brevis, adductor longus, adductor magnus, pectineus, and gracilis. They function to contract and pull the leg to the body's midline.

How many muscles are in the body? This is tricky to answer because each muscle is actually made of many layers of muscle tissue, and there are three types of muscle – skeletal, cardiac, and smooth. However, the commonly accepted answer is 650 skeletal muscles (the ones attached to bone).

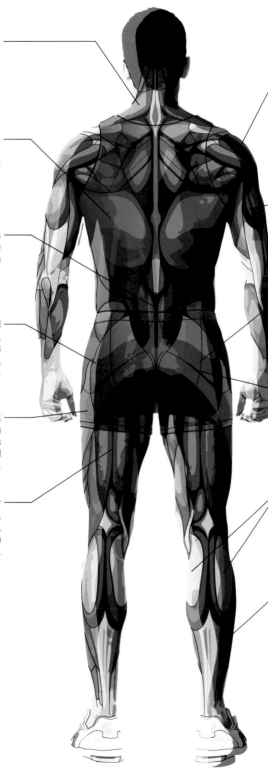

Trapezius – Resembling a trapezoid, it functions to move the scapula and support the arm.

Latissimus dorsi – The primary function of the broadest muscle of the back, also known as the "lat", is the adduction of the arm. It's often used when performing a pull-up or a chin-up.

Erector spinae – This bundle of muscles and tendons extends the length of the vertebral column. It functions to straighten the back and provide side-to-side rotation.

Abductors – Located in the buttocks and lateral hip region on both sides of the body, the abductors consist of the gluteus maximus, gluteus medius, gluteus minimus, and tensor fascia latae.

Iliotibial band – This is a longitudinal fibrous reinforcement of the tensor fascia latae. The action of the ITB and its associated muscles is to extend, abduct, and laterally rotate the hip.

Hamstrings – Consisting of three posterior thigh muscles, the semitendinosus, semimembranosus, and biceps femoris, hamstrings are responsible for knee flexion and hip extension.

Deltoids – The posterior, anterior, and lateral deltoid are primarily responsible for abduction of the arm on the frontal plane (lifting the arm up and out to the side).

Triceps brachii – This large muscle on the rear of the upper arm is principally responsible for extension of the elbow joint and straightening of the arm.

Gluteals – The gluteus maximus, gluteus medius, and gluteus minimus make up the buttocks. They're responsible for movement of the hip and thigh.

Piriformis – A pear-shaped muscle in the glute region that aids in external rotation of the hip. The piriformis laterally rotates the femur with hip extension and abducts the femur with hip flexion.

Gastrocnemius – These two heads of muscle run from just above the knee to the heel. Commonly called the calf, the gastrocnemius is essential for running and jumping.

Soleus – This powerful muscle in the rear portion of the lower leg works with the gastrocnemius to perform plantarflexion of the foot (pulling toes towards shins).

The 650 skeletal muscles are all named in Latin after their location, shape, function, or insertion and origin points. The hardest-working muscle in the body isn't shown here. It's the cardiac muscle – the heart – which beats once per second, or even faster during exercise or duress.

THE BIG SIX

In some shape or form, every exercise in this book takes its cues from the Big Six. These exercises are utilized on a nearly daily basis as you progress through the workouts in this book. The next few pages teach the benefits of each exercise, but above all provide tips and tricks for mastering form.

SQUATS

The squat doesn't work only the legs – it's a full-body exercise. Your hamstrings, quads, and glutes are, of course, the prime movers when you squat, but your core muscles also work to stabilize you.

CORRECT FORM

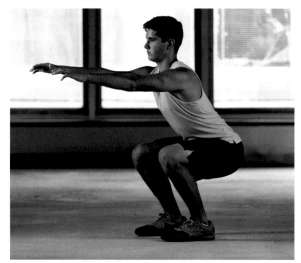

Keep your chest up, your glutes back, and your feet flat on the floor. Your back will arch slightly. The shins are close to vertical and the knees line up with the toes.

WHY SQUATS RULE

They Boost HGH and Testosterone
Squats increase muscle-building hormones throughout the entire body, causing a stimulus for growth.

They Improve Core Strength and Posture
Abdominals, back, and obliques must work to stabilize your spine and maintain an upright posture throughout the motion.

They Improve Hip Mobility
Deep squats work the hip through a larger range of motion, increasing hip mobility and flexibility, which may prevent back pain.

They Decrease the Risk of Injury
Building strength in the quads, glutes, hamstrings, lower back, and abs reduces your risk of injury when running, jumping, or changing direction.

They Increase Efficiency
Squats are a supercharger for the metabolic benefits of your workout.

They Increase Athletic Performance
Squats generate power, which will make you explosive on and off the field or court.

EVALUATING A SAFE DEPTH

Some people can't perform deep squats immediately due to hip dysfunction or weak or tight muscles. Here's how to establish the safe depth of your squats and to identify poor movement patterns or overcompensation.

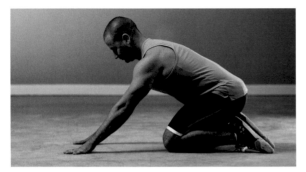

Face sideways on all fours in front of a mirror, core engaged and knees just wider than your shoulders. Drop your bottom down towards your feet and observe yourself.

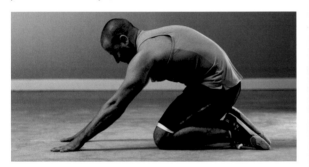

If your back looks rounded, you may have a weak or tight adductor magnus or glutes. When performing a squat, stop before your back gets round. It's okay to go shallow. As you progress through the book, your muscles will strengthen and hip mobility will increase. You can then squat more deeply.

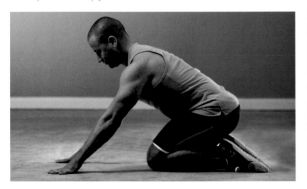

If your back looks flat, you will be able to perform a good, deep squat with moderate depth.

HIP DYSFUNCTION

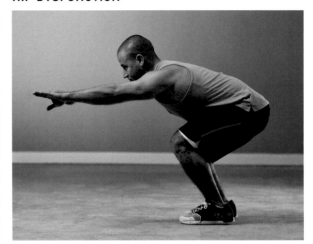

If you tip forwards while squatting, you have weak glutes, which are the primary muscle used in hip extension. You're tipping because your lower back is switching on to compensate. Squat less deeply. Progress through the book and your muscles will strengthen so you can squat lower.

ANKLE DORSIFLECTION

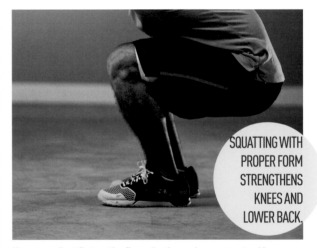

SQUATTING WITH PROPER FORM STRENGTHENS KNEES AND LOWER BACK.

Keep your feet flat on the floor: As shown above, correct ankle dorsiflexion (pulling the feet and toes back towards the shin) is about 15 degrees. Lack of flexibility in the calves and soleus, or wearing bulky trainers, can cause lost mobility in the ankles. Lack of dorsiflexion can lead to several issues when you squat; the easiest to spot and correct is the heels lifting off the floor. You'll improve flexibility by progressing through the book; more flexibility will also enhance any athletic move that involves landing and decelerating the body.

LUNGES

Lunges prepare the body for deceleration and change of direction. Any weaknesses could lead to overcompensation, decreased performance, and possibly injury.

As you perform a lunge, focus on moving your torso only up and down, not pushing it forwards. This keeps your weight balanced evenly through the front foot, allowing you to dig the front heel down and back to perform the movement. Press into the floor with your heel, which tones more lower-body muscle.

These key points ensure perfect, pain-free lunges.

CORRECT FORM

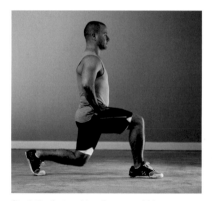

Stack the feet, ankles, knees, and hips on top of one another, and step straight back, keeping them in line. Keep the chest up, and the shin of the front leg relatively vertical.

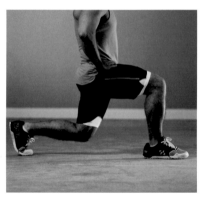

Keep the trailing knee underneath the hips to load the hip, utilizing the front leg glute to perform the majority of the work.

WATCH OUT FOR THESE FLAWS

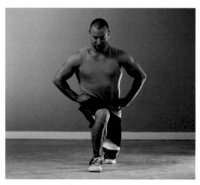

Don't let the knees cave in, and keep the hips forwards at all times.

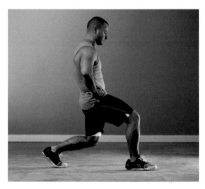

The trailing hip should not sink or dip.

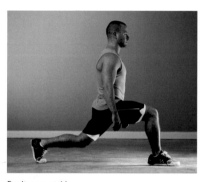

Don't over-stride ...

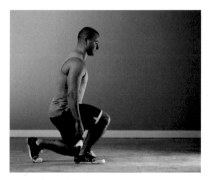

... or under-stride.

CORRECT FORM

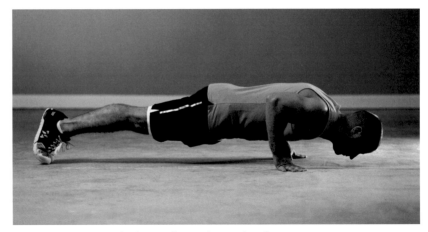

Keep elbows above wrists, hands rotated outwards approximately to 45 degrees. Tighten your core, and keep the pelvis in a posterior pelvic tilt – imagine wearing a belt and pulling the buckle up towards your navel.

PRESS-UPS

The press-up may be the perfect multi-muscle (compound) exercise, effective at building strength and stability and burning body fat.

Most people associate press-ups with the chest, arms, and/or back, which is correct since the primary movers are the triceps, pectorals, serratus anterior, and lats. What most people forget, though, is that the press-up is a "moving plank", and abdominal muscles dominate when it comes to spinal stability during press-ups. The rectus abdominis is the primary stabilizer for preventing your hips sagging, while the obliques prevent lateral shifting and twisting.

STARTING POSITION

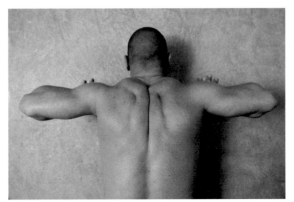

Incorrect starting position: People often set up with their hand position shoulder high and elbow width to make the exercise easier. Viewed from above, this looks like the letter T.

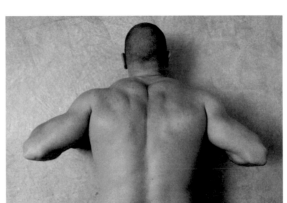

Correct starting position: The arms should form an angle of 20–40 degrees from the body. Viewed from above, you'll look like an arrow. This is easier on the shoulder joint and leads to higher activation of the pectorals and triceps.

BURPEES

Done correctly, the Burpee might be the best metabolic-boosting exercise on the planet, an incredible total body strength and cardiovascular exercise.

The Burpee has four athletic components: a squat, a martial arts or wrestling style sprawl as the legs hop back, a press-up, and a vertical leap. The key to successfully completing a Burpee is to break it down into these parts.

START SLOW. PERFECT EACH STAGE, THEN ADD SPEED AND REPS.

CORRECT FORM

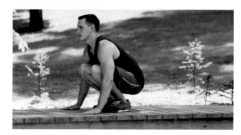

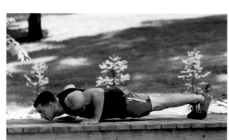

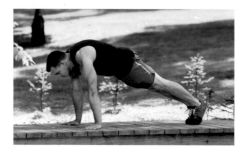

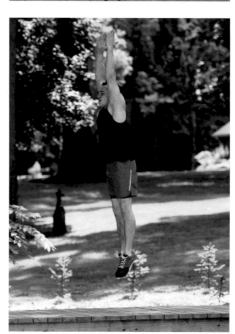

01 **Squat:** The final phase of the squat should look like a sitting frog. You'll also return to this position before the vertical jump. Hip mobility often inhibits jumping the feet far enough forwards to have heels on the floor. Make sure to rock your weight back into your heels and lift your chest.

02 **Sprawl:** This extends the legs and positions you in a plank. Don't jump too far – arms at 90 degrees, palms level with chest, and shoulders over wrists. Don't sag – engage your core and use a posterior pelvic tilt to lock it in.

03 **Press-up:** This is where I see the greatest number of flaws during Burpees. You should not sprawl all the way to the floor with no control, "bounce" your chest off the floor, or lift your chest and arch like a cobra.

04 **Leap:** Always start the leap from the squat position. This stable platform allows you to drive through the lower body and propel yourself into the air. While in the air, make sure to achieve "triple extension", which means you've fully extended not just the arms, but the ankles, the knees, and the hips. Getting into triple extension requires starting from a bent position, in which all joints are primed for movement.

CORRECT FORM

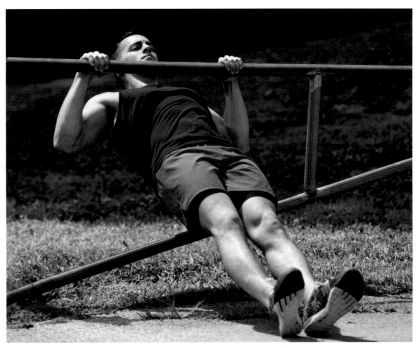

INVERTED ROWS

Think of inverted rows as the counter-punch to the press-up. They utilize all the pulling muscles, opposite those used during a press-up.

Inverted rows work biceps, lats, traps, and deltoids. They're essential for creating balance and symmetry in the body.

All inverted row variations require you to keep your body in an elevated horizontal inverted plank. Maintaining elevated hips in this way fires the glutes and hamstrings, and your abdominals stabilize the spine. Your key focus is to squeeze the shoulder blades and lift the chest to the bar.

FIXING FLAWS

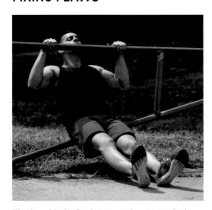

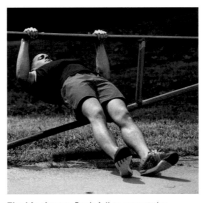

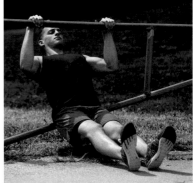

The head bob: Don't jut out the chin to find an extra centimetre or two of motion. A failure to retract the shoulder blades misses the entire purpose of an inverted row. Instead, keep the chin slightly forwards and down, and the neck aligned with the cervical vertebrae.

The hip thrust: Don't fail to retract the scapulae, let the elbows drift behind the body, or jerk your forearm to get halfway up and thrust your crotch to the heavens. Instead, squeeze the glutes, engage the core, and use a posterior pelvic tilt to help lock in the core.

The sag: Don't let hips sag or glutes drop. This indicates a lack of strength in the glutes, hamstrings, pelvic floor, and core. To build strength and work up to a horizontal inverted plank, bend legs, place feet flat on the ground, and engage the glutes and core for stability.

CORRECT FORM

PULL-UPS

Most of us spend large amounts of time sitting at a desk, and this leads to the devolution of the body. Pull-ups build incredible strength and posture, and also decompress the spine.

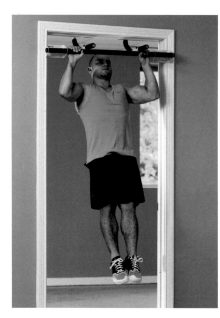

Despite popular belief, pull-ups aren't vertical; you should move up and back.

Pack the shoulders and brace the core by assuming a hollow body hold position with your feet slightly forwards of your hips. Tighten the glutes to unload the spine. Look at the bar, keeping the chin up. Pull backwards, squeezing the shoulder blades and engaging the lats, lifting as if trying to touch your chest to the bar. Lower slowly, with control.

These points apply to both overhand pull-ups and underhand chin-ups.

ACHIEVING MORE MOBILITY

Correct mobility is essential to completing any exercise, but it's absolutely critical when undertaking pull-ups. Before performing pull-ups, begin with a drill to open the shoulders and chest and create mobility to hang correctly. You'll need a foam roller and a towel.

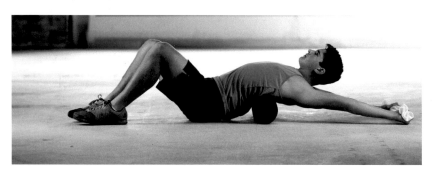

01 Place the foam roller directly below the shoulder blades, lift the hips, and extend the arms, keeping the towel taut, the backs of your hands on the floor, shoulders packed, and elbows locked.

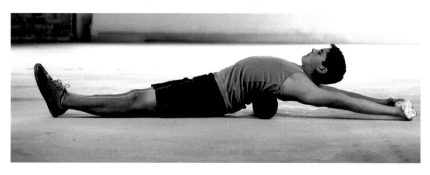

02 When ready, extend your legs and your lower back to the floor without elevating hands or bending arms.

DEAD HANG

Now that you're mobile, the next step is to get comfortable hanging. The genesis of any pull-up is the dead hang. A strong grip equals a strong upper body. Get comfortable hanging from the bar but make sure you keep correct form with your shoulders packed.

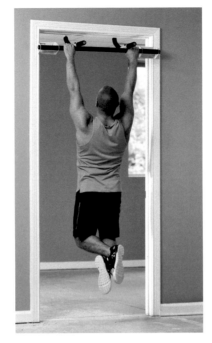

Shoulders packed: Think of the dead hang as a hanging plank. Just like a plank, it's all about keeping your shoulders down, ribcage down and in, core engaged, and glutes tight.

FIXING FLAWS

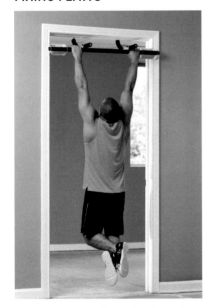

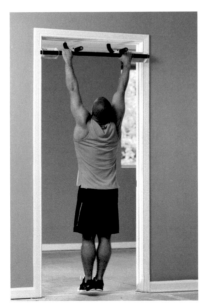

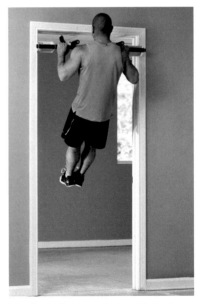

Shoulders by ears: If your shoulders look like this, practise the hanging scapula retraction found in Level 1 until this position becomes comfortable for you.

Chin up: The simplest trick for great pull-ups is keeping your chin up. By so doing, you'll lengthen your body and position it to maximize your results on the bar.

Lean back: Squeeze and engage the back muscles, and at the top of the motion lean slightly back as if touching chest to bar. This allows the the large back muscles to activate.

MODIFICATIONS

Almost every exercise can be made more or less challenging with some fundamental modifications. This allows you to quickly and easily adapt an exercise to meet your ability level. These pages show how to apply each modification to a press-up, but it's possible to perform them on any exercise.

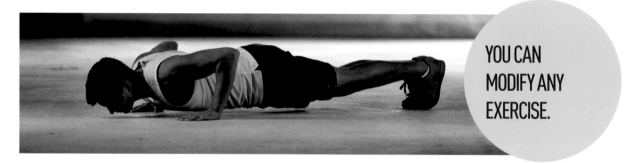

YOU CAN MODIFY ANY EXERCISE.

BODY ANGLE

Adjusting the angle between your body and the floor allows you to shift more or less weight onto the working muscles.

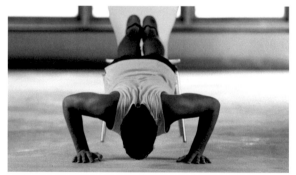

More difficult: Elevating the feet makes the exercise more challenging by transferring weight to the upper body, which then has to work harder.

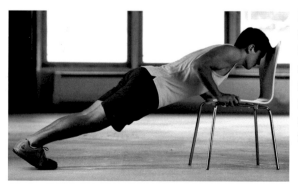

Less difficult: The work of a press-up is performed by the chest, back, and shoulders. With the hands elevated on a chair, bench, or other prop, your weight shifts from the upper body to the lower body.

STABILITY

Stability is the constant fight between your body's centre of gravity and its contact with the floor – its base of support. Simply raising one foot off of the floor decreases stability and makes an exercise more challenging. Stability-based modifications improve core and joint strength, making you more athletic and decreasing the risk of injury.

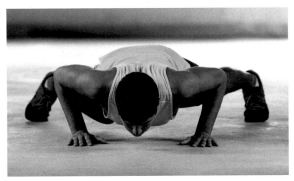

More difficult: Touching fingers and thumbs in the shape of a diamond directly under your chest narrows the base of support and decreases stability.

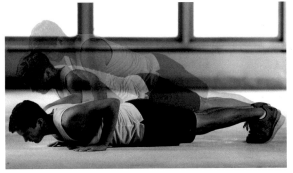

Less difficult: By opening either the feet or hands, you widen the base of support and make the exercise easier because your weight is distributed over a larger area.

RANGE OF MOTION

In a full range of motion (ROM), you perform an exercise from the absolute top point to the absolute bottom point and back again. Changing the ROM by shortening, lengthening, or even stopping can make the exercise easier or harder.

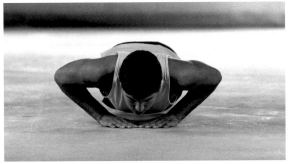

More difficult: Performing a greater amount of work on each rep during the toughest part of the exercise increases the challenge. Lower; then come up only halfway, lower fully again, and go fully up. You've performed 1.5 reps.

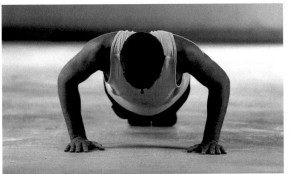

Less difficult: Half press-ups, in which you lower your body only halfway, decrease the ROM – a good way to build confidence in the early stages of practising a new exercise.

POINTS OF CONTACT

The more points of contact you have with the floor, the easier the exercise. With fewer contact points, you have to move the same mass with fewer joints.

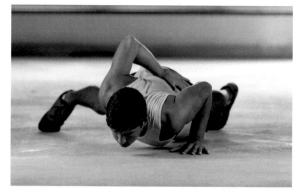

More difficult: Raising an arm off of the floor decreases the number of joints from four to three, increases the load on the working arm, and decreases stability.

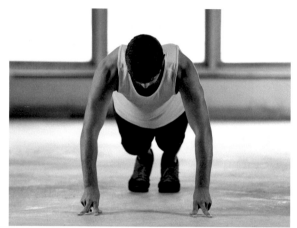

Even more difficult: The surface area of the points of contact also plays a role in modifying the exercise. Going from the entire palm on the floor to a two-finger press-up decreases the surface area.

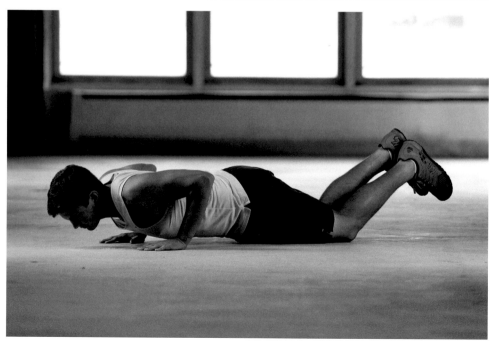

Less difficult: Dropping the knees to the floor inclines and shortens the body, increasing stability and decreasing the amount of mass moved during the press-up.

SPEED

Altering the speed of an exercise can make it easier or harder. To know the speed of an exercise, though, you must understand the different types of muscle contraction, as each relates to the speed.

TYPES OF MUSCLE CONTRACTION

Concentric contractions: When a muscle is activated and required to lift a load, it begins to shorten. Contractions that permit the muscle to shorten are called concentric contractions. Bicep curls are a concentric contraction, but for the speed modification, think of them as acceleration.

Eccentric contractions: An eccentric contraction increases tension on a muscle as it lengthens. Eccentric contractions usually occur when the muscle opposes a stronger force, causing it to lengthen as it contracts. An example is the lowering phase of a squat. Think of eccentric contractions as controlled movements similar to decelerating or braking while at high speed.

Isometric contractions: In this type of contraction, the muscle is activated, but instead of being shortened or lengthened, it's held. Think of it as a racing car driver with the engine at peak revs but clutch balanced waiting for the green light. Isometric contractions can also form a pause at the mid-point of an exercise.

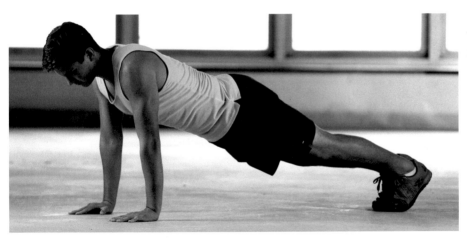

Hold the start position: This forces you to defy gravity and hold an isometric contraction while you build strength in your core and shoulders.

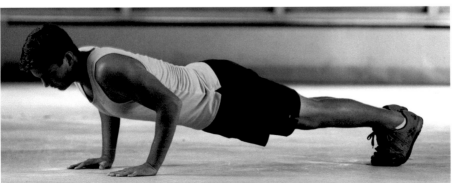

Slow the lowering phase: Taking four seconds to lower to the deepest part of the press-up and then pressing back up to the starting position makes the chest, shoulders, and triceps contract eccentrically.

FUNCTIONAL WARM-UPS

Functional training is a classification of exercise that involves training the body for activities performed in daily life.

For example, squats equate to getting in and out of a chair, and pull-ups hark back to the survival skills necessary for early humans, who had to pull themselves into the higher branches of trees to evade predators.

It's not that exercise such as power lifting isn't functional per se, but unless you're a fireman or in an occupation that requires lifting or moving heavy objects off of a trapped person, or a sumo wrestler, you probably won't be moving large amounts of mass on a daily basis.

A functional exercise should prepare us for a daily activity or mimic a movement used in everyday life. Functional training should make you more stable, balanced, and confident in performing these motions.

The next five exercises can be performed independently or chained together to form a cyclical yoga-inspired flow. The goal of each is to increase mobility and balance, and prepare your body for the challenges ahead.

Performing an exercise like the L-sit chin-up requires core and shoulder strength and mobility – especially hip mobility. Performing the functional warm-ups will not only help you move better, it will also increase performance and help prevent injury.

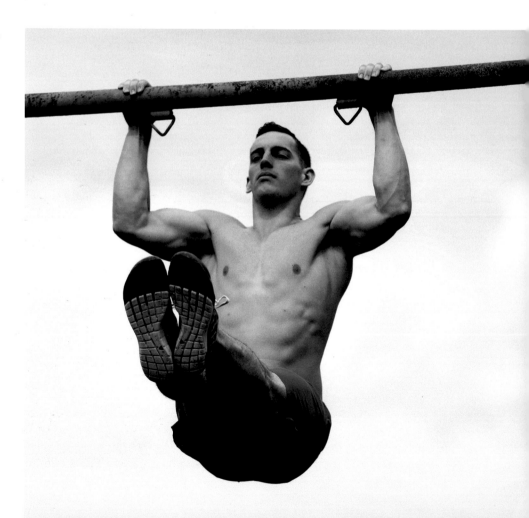

INLINE LUNGE

As a functional warm-up, the inline lunge activates the glutes, quads, and hamstrings. It also forces you to engage your core and challenges your proprioception – your unconscious ability to perceive movement and spatial orientation, which arises from stimuli within the body.

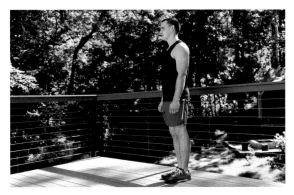

01 Stand tall with feet hip-width apart and arms at your sides. Activate your core and glutes.

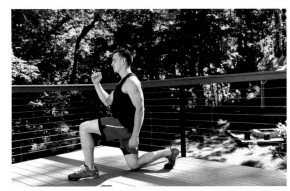

02 Take a step forwards with one leg, bend both legs, and lower into a lunge position. Attempt to place the toes of the rear foot in line with the front heel and knee, as if standing on an invisible tight rope.

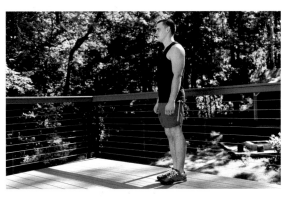

03 Straighten both legs, pressing them firmly into the floor. Alternate legs. Perform five lunges per leg, for a total of 10 reps.

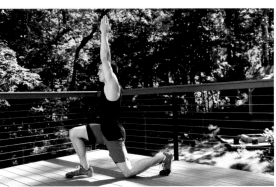

Variation
For an added balance challenge, try extending the arms overhead during the lunge. This will require, and in turn result in, greater trunk stability.

RESTING SQUAT

Since the dawn of time, our ancestors knew the power of resting squats. Human beings have crouched all the way down into these to perform activities like working or cooking over a fire, and for relaxing. The sitting squat will help to open your hips and provide dorsiflexion in the ankles and feet, preparing you for squats.

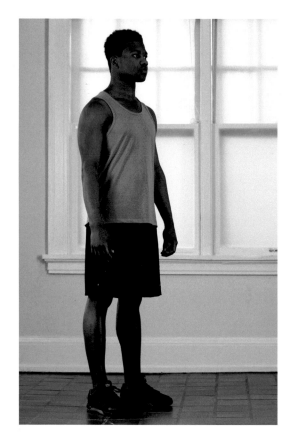

01 Stand tall with feet approximately shoulder-width apart and arms hanging by your sides.

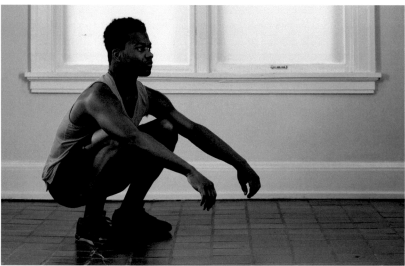

02 Bend at the knees and lower until your glutes are resting on the back of your calves. Do not let your heels lift off of the floor. Keep your chest up and hold this position for 30 seconds before standing. Repeat three to five times.

TRUNK STABILITY PRESS-UP

Without adequate stability in the trunk, you waste energy, resulting in poor performance and increasing your risk of injury. The trunk stability press-up helps strengthen and stabilize the spine and trunk during a closed-chain upper-body movement – one where the upper body is fixed in place against an immobile surface.

PLACE HANDS/ THUMBS LEVEL WITH CHIN TO MAKE IT EASIER.

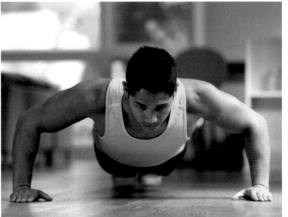

01 Lie on your stomach with your hands shoulder-width apart and thumbs level with your forehead. Raise onto your toes and lift your torso from the ground.

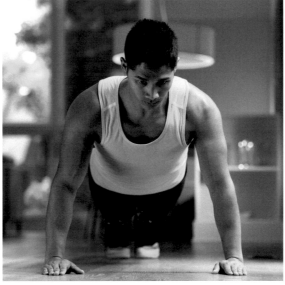

02 Maintaining a rigid torso, lift yourself as a unit into a press-up position, making sure the lumbar spine does not dip down.

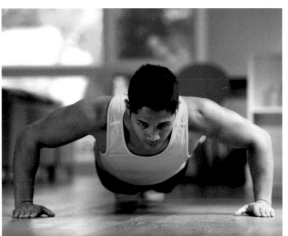

03 Lower back down into the same position as in step 1. Perform three to five reps with correct form.

INNER THIGH MOBILITY

Performance is compromised by poor joint mobility. The greater your joint mobility, the greater your ROM, and the more kinetic energy/tension – and therefore power – you'll be able to generate. Warm up the hips and groin with this simple yet incredibly effective inner thigh mobility stretch.

ENGAGE CORE IN ALL PHASES.

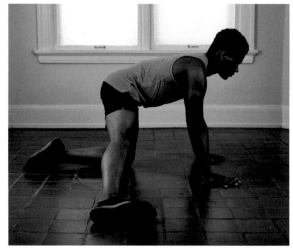

01 Begin on your hands and knees with your back flat, and straighten your right leg out to the side until it is perpendicular to your torso.

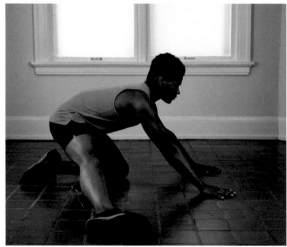

02 Keep your back flat and push your hips back as far as possible.

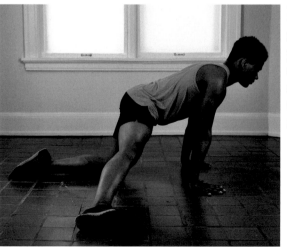

03 Push your hips forwards as far as you can, keeping your back flat and arms straight. Return to the starting position to complete one rep. Perform eight reps on each leg.

THORACIC ROTATION

Improve your posture by increasing the mobility in your thoracic spine. It's especially beneficial for those who spend a lot of time at a desk or keyboard or spend too much time bench pressing at the gym.

DON'T "FLAP" ELBOW.

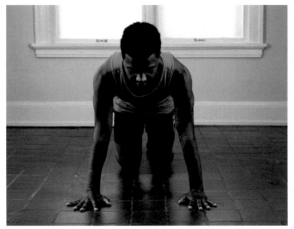

01 Begin on your hands and knees, with a flat back and straight arms.

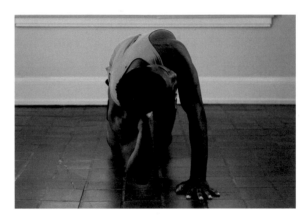

02 Bring your right hand behind your head and rotate your right elbow in towards the floor. Make sure to rotate through the thoracic spine and trunk rather than through the arm.

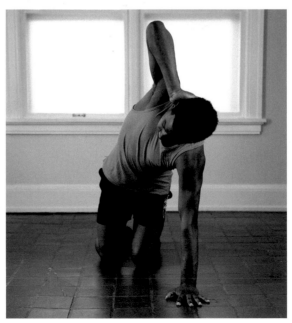

03 Rotate the right elbow outwards to the ceiling, opening the chest and rotating your head and upper back as far as you can. Rotate back inwards and repeat for eight reps, then switch sides.

RECOVERY

Bodyweight workouts require you to exert great stress upon your body. Afterwards, your muscles will be tired and sore. Recovery practices are critical for injury prevention and consistent training, and they enable you to give maximum effort for maximum results. Make these four simple practices part of your regular post-workout routine.

1 STRETCH

Stretching isn't sexy and doesn't make you look good without a shirt, but it's the most underrated aspect of athletic development.

Without the necessary flexibility and muscle pliability, you'll struggle to find the depth required to maximize your ability to burn calories and build new muscle.

- Run through all of the exercises found in the Functional Warm-ups pages post-workout as well as pre-workout to increase your flexibility and mobility.

2 FOAM ROLL

The fascia is connective tissue that wraps around the muscles in the body. It can become tense or constricted while working out, causing pain.

You can massage yourself with a foam roller to relieve muscle tightness. This is called self-myofacial release.

- Perform foam rolling, a key component of recovery. See Foam-Rolling Technique.

FOAM-ROLLING TECHNIQUE

Use a foam roller to "roll out" the muscles as a warm-up, after working out, or whenever you feel pain. This alleviates soreness and stiffness, promotes circulation of oxygenated blood, and even breaks up scar tissue and restrictions in the fascia.

A foam roller also allows you to apply targeted pressure to specific spots in the muscle that may be causing pain.

Look for a high-density foam roller that's about 7.5cm (3in) in diameter. You can find them at sports equipment shops or online.

The basic technique is the same, regardless of whether you use it on the legs, back, or arms. There's a lot of freedom for experimentation when using the roller. See what works well and feels best for you, and manipulate the roller to the correct position. You can create your own techniques to meet your needs.

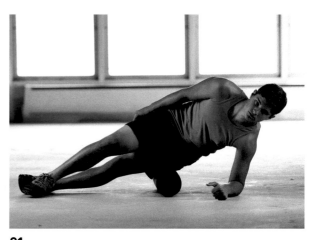

01 Position your body on the roller. The weight of your body will apply pressure on your muscles. Roll back and forth slowly. When you find a tender spot in the area you're working, pause and wait for the discomfort to diminish. This could take up to one minute and may be uncomfortable.

3 SLEEP

Sleep is the necessary downtime your body needs to restore itself.

Other mammals don't willingly delay sleep the way we humans do. Sacrificing hours of sleep over a long period of time can negatively impact your mental strength and commitment to training sessions. Another drawback of not getting enough rest at night is that you'll want to eat more than you need to. Leptin is a hormone that regulates appetite, and its levels fall in the bodies of people who haven't had enough rest, increasing food cravings.

If you find it difficult to get to sleep, make sure to cut out caffeinated beverages. One of the many benefits of regular exercise is that it can help you fall asleep faster, and it contributes to sounder, deeper sleep. But don't exercise right before you go to bed, because that may have the opposite effect. It could get you wired and make it harder to get to sleep.

- Sleep at least seven hours; note that many athletes may need up to nine hours.

4 ICE

Intense exercise causes microtrauma, or tiny tears, in muscle fibres.

This sounds scary, but it's a good thing because micro tears stimulate muscle-cell activity, helping repair the damage and actually strengthening the muscles. Applying ice helps the body recover faster and reduces muscle pain and soreness after intense training sessions.

Ice constricts blood vessels and flushes waste products out of the affected tissue. It decreases metabolic activity and slows down physiological processes. And it reduces swelling and tissue breakdown. Afterwards, the body has to warm itself, resulting in increased blood flow that improves the healing process.

- Fill your tub with water 12–15°C (53–59°F) and submerge your body for 10–15 minutes to gain the maximum benefit.

- Or instead of an ice bath, apply localized ice (for example bags of frozen peas) to specific areas of the body for 10–15 minutes. Don't apply these directly to the skin; wrap them in a towel first.

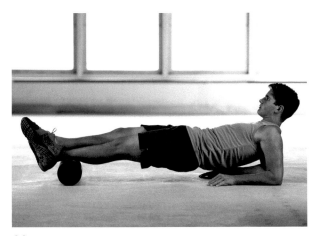

02 When the area is no longer sensitive, roll up or down the muscle on the roller. When you identify any other sensitive spots, again pause and wait for the discomfort to diminish.

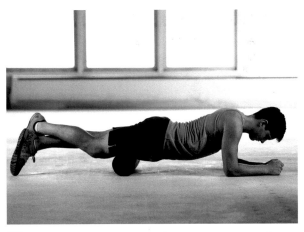

03 When tender areas can be rolled over without pain, continue rolling regularly to keep the area relaxed.

NUTRITION

Bodyweight exercises are all about moving your own mass; the heavier you are, the harder it will be. So it's essential to prioritize nutrition to become a lean, mean performance machine.

Exercise effectively tears and breaks apart muscle fibres. Protein is essential for exercise because it contains amino acids, the building block of new muscle. Since it repairs muscle, you must provide the body a constant supply of protein throughout the entire day for optimum muscle growth. Having a body with lean muscle mass fuelled by protein has another benefit in that it decreases body fat percentage.

What about carbs? Aren't they the devil? The key is to save them for post-workout meals, when your body uses the simple sugars and starches to replace those energy stores. Whole grains, fruits, and vegetables are the best carbohydrates to consume while following the programmes in this book – keep it to around 100g a day.

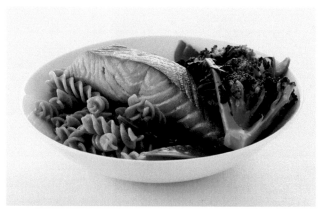

An excellent post-workout meal: With about 23g of protein per serving, salmon paired with whole-wheat pasta or quinoa and nutrient-packed broccoli and mangetout helps repair and replenish the body.

PROTEIN: HOW MUCH DO YOU NEED, AND HOW CAN YOU GET IT?

To calculate how much protein to eat while on a bodyweight exercise regimen, multiply your weight in pounds by between 0.9 and 1.1. The result gives you the number of grams of protein you need daily.

Daily protein requirement for a 10-stone man	126–154g	Daily protein requirement for a 13-stone man	162–198g	Daily protein requirement for a 16-stone man	198–242g
Sample meal plan	**Protein**	**Sample meal plan**	**Protein**	**Sample meal plan**	**Protein**
Extra large egg	7g	All of the protein for a 10 stone man plus:		All of the protein for a 13-stone man plus:	
2 tbsp peanut butter	7g	85g bacon	10g	170g rump steak	52g
170g tuna	52g	85g cottage cheese	10.5g		
170g black beans	15g	125g tofu	10g		
2 slices Swiss cheese, such as Emmental	15g				
85g chicken drumstick	23g		30.5g		52g
180g cannellini beans	20g		+		+
100g Greek yoghurt	10g		149g		179.5g
	149g		**179.5g**		**231.5g**

NUTRITION BLUEPRINT

Six simple steps create a solid nutritional foundation.

- Eat four to six small meals each day: breakfast, lunch, and dinner, with high-protein mid-morning, mid-afternoon, and early-evening snacks.
- Avoid sugar and processed foods.
- Limit carbohydrates to unprocessed complex carbs, such as sweet potatoes.
- Eliminate fizzy drinks, sweetened coffee beverages, and other high-calorie sugary drinks, including sports drinks.
- Cut out alcohol.
- Drink lots of water – it flushes toxins and keeps you feeling satiated.

GREAT POST-WORKOUT SNACKS AND MEALS

These small meals are perfect for a man on a bodyweight workout regimen because they include both proteins and carbs.

- A protein shake with milk and a banana
- Half an avocado stuffed with cottage cheese
- Spinach salad topped with grilled chicken
- A banana sliced lengthwise and spread with nut butter

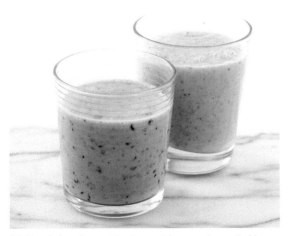

Drinking shakes that contain whey protein can make you feel less hungry later, and helps you lose body fat and better preserve muscle mass.

HYDRATION

During exercise, you may lose up to 2 litres of water an hour. Just a 2 per cent decrease in weight caused by dehydration can lead to a 20 per cent decrease in athletic performance. For every litre of fluid lost, core temperature increases, heart rate rises, glycogen stored in muscles is used more rapidly, and lactic acid increases.

HOW MUCH SHOULD YOU DRINK?

What's the ideal amount to consume when pursuing the programmes in this book? The daily amount of water intake will differ from person to person and will vary based on activity.

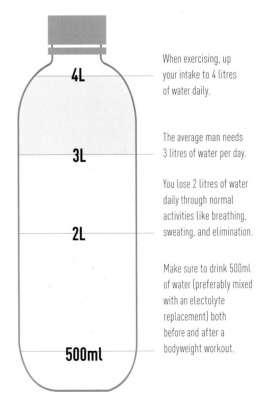

4L — When exercising, up your intake to 4 litres of water daily.

3L — The average man needs 3 litres of water per day.

You lose 2 litres of water daily through normal activities like breathing, sweating, and elimination.

2L —

Make sure to drink 500ml of water (preferably mixed with an electrolyte replacement) both before and after a bodyweight workout.

500ml —

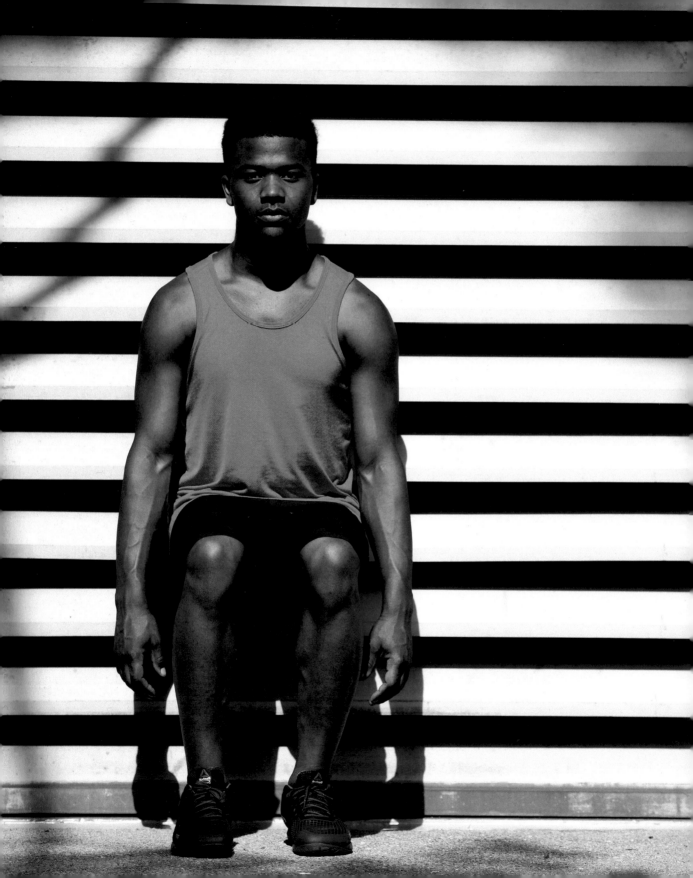

LEVEL

1

Level 1 provides you with a thorough understanding of foundation exercises such as squats, press-ups, and pull-ups, each with options to make them more or less challenging. These exercises focus on building strength, muscle tone, and definition, while teaching the base forms required to quickly progress to higher levels.

DEAD HANG

This is a great introduction to bodyweight training because it teaches body awareness and helps you develop the fundamental grip strength vital in all hanging exercises.

MORE DIFFICULT

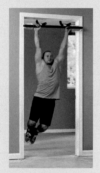

Modify stability: In step 2, gently swing your body from side to side to perform dead swings. This will force you to recruit the muscles in your core for stabilization.

LESS DIFFICULT

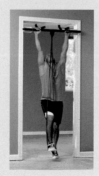

Modify stability: Use a resistance band, or place one foot on a chair, to provide support and stability while you build confidence and strength.

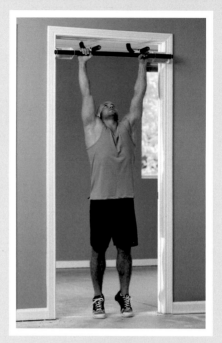

01 Stand directly under your pull-up bar.

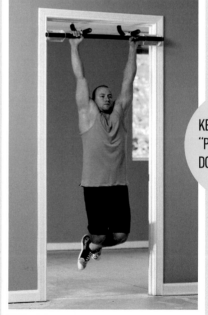

KEEP SHOULDERS "PACKED" – PULLED DOWN AND BACK.

02 Hop up and grab the bar with an overhand grip (palms facing away) wider than your shoulders, and hang from the bar with straight arms. Try to hang with good form for as long as possible.

MOUNTAIN CLIMBER

A challenging cardiovascular exercise, mountain climbers mimic finding a foothold while climbing a summit and work your core, hip flexors, and legs.

MORE DIFFICULT

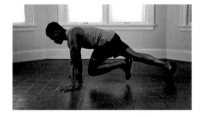

Modify range of motion and reps: During step 2, extend partially, then add a second pull of the knee to the chest before switching legs.

LESS DIFFICULT

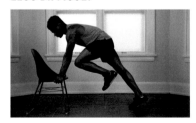

Modify body angle: For all steps, elevate your hands on a prop, shifting weight to the lower body so it's easier to sustain the plank.

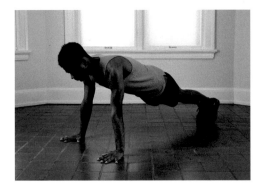

01 Position your hands on the floor slightly wider than your shoulders. Rise up onto your toes, and engage the core to form a straight back and balance your weight between your toes and head. This is the plank position.

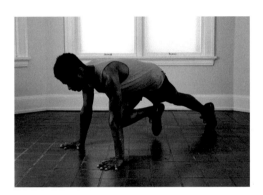

02 Bending your right leg, pull your knee in towards your chest while keeping your core engaged.

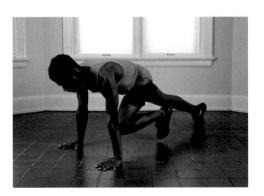

03 Straighten the right leg back into its original position and simultaneously pull the left knee towards the chest. Repeat, alternating leg positions, with controlled speed.

ELBOWS STRAIGHT, MAINTAIN A RIGID PLANK POSITION THROUGHOUT.

REVERSE PLANK BRIDGE

Create stability and balance through the back side with this simple bodyweight staple.

MORE DIFFICULT

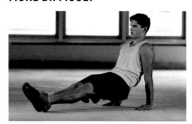

Modify reps: Add a small pulse to step 2 by lowering halfway down and then re-engaging the core and glutes to perform 1.5 reps, then repeat.

LESS DIFFICULT

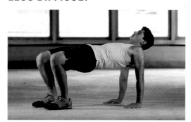

Modify speed and points of contact: In all steps, bend your knees to decrease the length of the body.

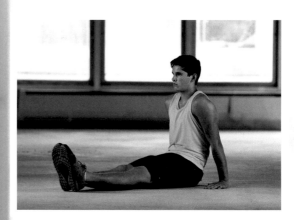

01 Sit on the floor with your legs extended in front of you. Place your palms on the floor with fingers slightly spread and pointing towards your toes.

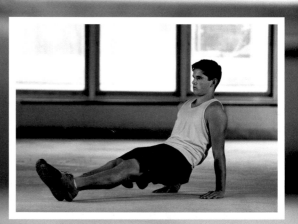

02 Press into your palms and lift your hips and torso towards the ceiling.

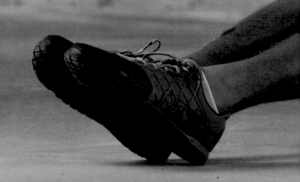

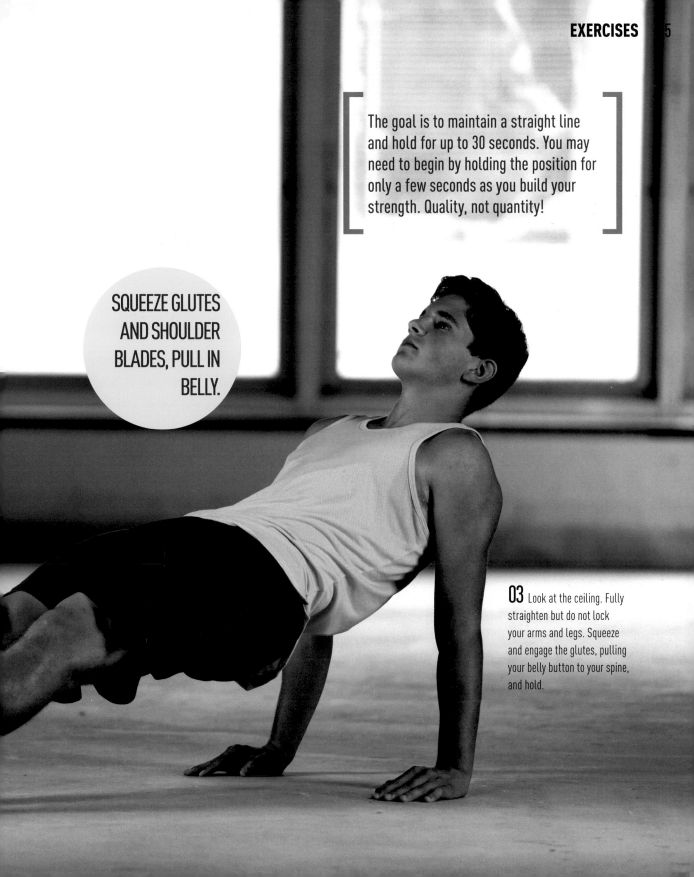

The goal is to maintain a straight line and hold for up to 30 seconds. You may need to begin by holding the position for only a few seconds as you build your strength. Quality, not quantity!

SQUEEZE GLUTES AND SHOULDER BLADES, PULL IN BELLY.

03 Look at the ceiling. Fully straighten but do not lock your arms and legs. Squeeze and engage the glutes, pulling your belly button to your spine, and hold.

ALTERNATING LATERAL LUNGE

Lateral lunges strengthen and tone the glutes, hamstrings, and thighs. In the process, they increase dynamic balance.

MORE DIFFICULT

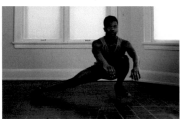

Modify stability and range of motion: In all steps, elevate the bending leg to decrease your stability and require greater activation of the glutes, quads, and hamstrings.

LESS DIFFICULT

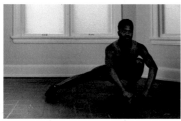

Modify stability: Throughout the exercise, perform all reps to the same side to increase stability, allowing you to build confidence and focus on depth.

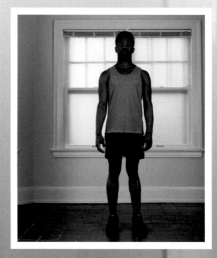

01 Stand tall with feet shoulder-width apart and toes pointing forwards.

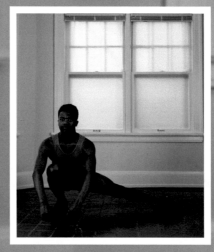

02 Step out to the right side (laterally) away from the body. Remain tall and keep your weight in the heel as you push back your hips, lowering your body until the thigh is parallel to the floor.

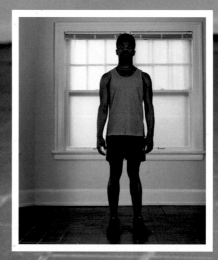

03 Push back off of the bent leg, straightening the hips and knee to return to your starting position.

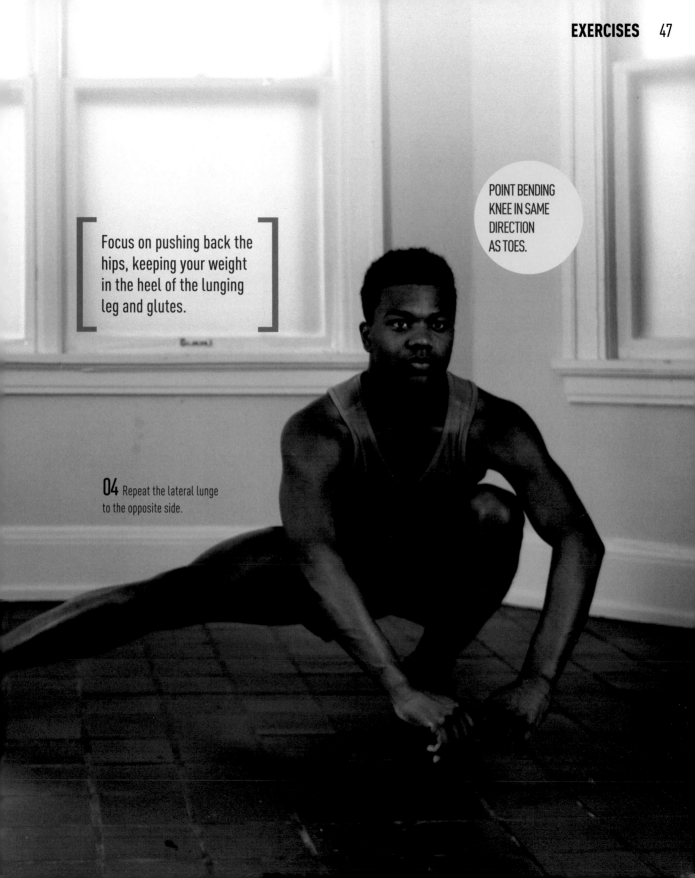

POINT BENDING
KNEE IN SAME
DIRECTION
AS TOES.

Focus on pushing back the
hips, keeping your weight
in the heel of the lunging
leg and glutes.

04 Repeat the lateral lunge
to the opposite side.

STANDARD PRESS-UP

Done correctly, press-ups build upper body and core strength, using the muscles of the chest, back, shoulders, triceps, abs, and even the legs.

MORE DIFFICULT

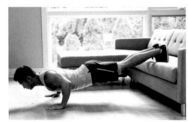

Modify body angle: In all steps, elevate your feet on a box or bench to decline your body, transferring weight into the upper body to cause it to work harder.

LESS DIFFICULT

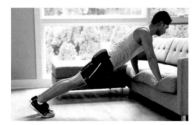

Modify body angle: Elevate your hands on a prop to transfer more of the load away from the arms and shoulders and to the lower body,

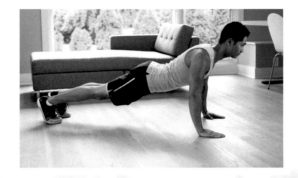

01 Begin with arms straight, your weight balanced on hands and toes. This is the plank position.

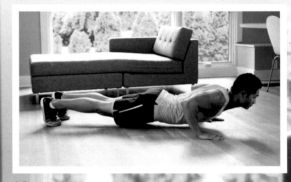

02 Bend your elbows, bringing your chest towards the floor. Your elbows should bend slightly beyond 90 degrees.

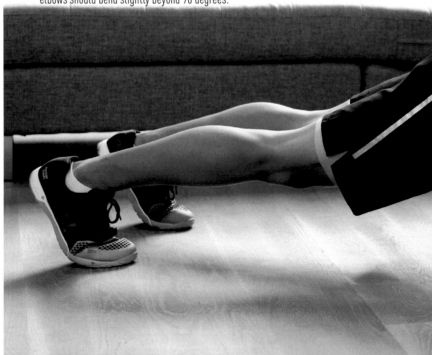

When performing a standard press-up, imagine a wooden rod along your entire back. The rod should remain in contact with your heels, hips, and upper back at all times.

LEGS, HIPS, AND BACK SHOULD BE STRAIGHT.

Try this ...

There are many variations to the standard press-up. Adjust your hand position to work slightly different muscle groups.

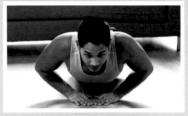

HEART TO HANDS PRESS-UP
Place both hands on the floor below the sternum. You primarily work the triceps in this variation, also called a diamond press-up.

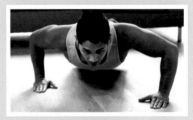

STAGGERED PRESS-UP
With its hands at different heights along the body, this variation decreases stability and helps strengthen the serratus anterior.

03 Push up through your palms, straightening your arms to return to the starting position. Repeat steps 2 and 3 as described.

CHIN-UP

Chin-ups are a bodyweight training essential because they work the biceps, back, and core while supercharging your metabolism.

MORE DIFFICULT

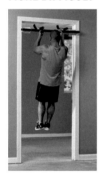

Modify speed: In step 3, lower slowly, straightening arms over a count of four to produce an eccentric muscle contraction that builds strength.

LESS DIFFICULT

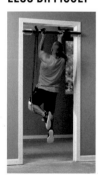

Modify points of contact and stability: For all steps, use a resistance band or place your foot on a chair to assist the chin-up by adding leverage.

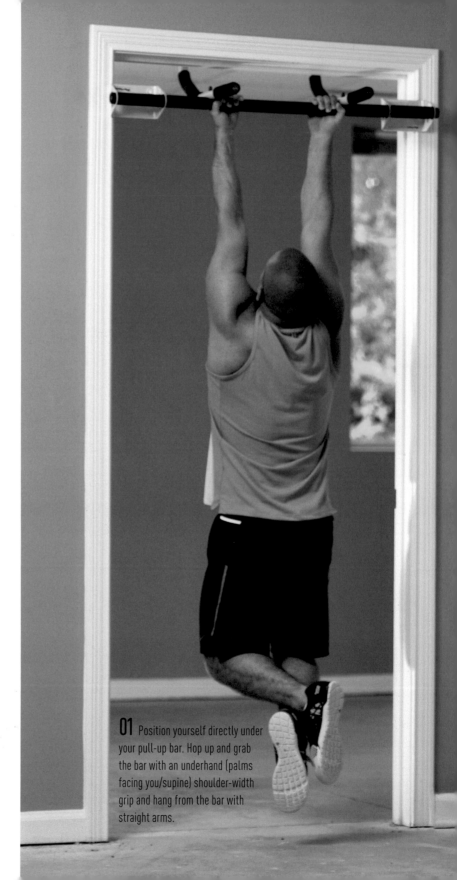

01 Position yourself directly under your pull-up bar. Hop up and grab the bar with an underhand (palms facing you/supine) shoulder-width grip and hang from the bar with straight arms.

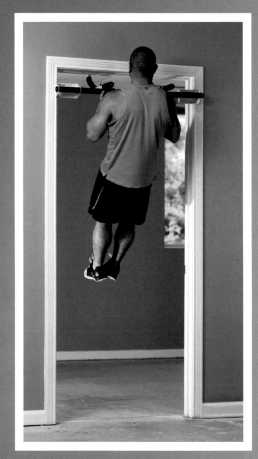

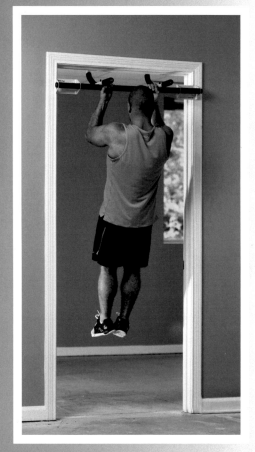

02 Pull yourself up until your chin is above the bar. Pause.

03 Lower yourself down with control. Repeat steps 2 and 3 as described.

ISOLATE BACK, SQUEEZE BICEPS. DON'T SWING!

Chin-ups are slightly easier than pull-ups because the supine position of the hands allows for greater activation of the biceps.

CLOSE-GRIP INVERTED ROW

This exercise dedicated to the back will build bullet-proof shoulders and aid in injury prevention.

MORE DIFFICULT

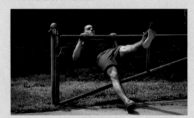

Modify stability and range of motion: Raise a foot to decrease stability and challenge the core. Switch feet halfway through the reps.

LESS DIFFICULT

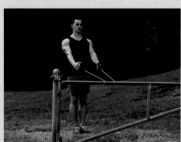

Modify stability and points of contact: Perform this exercise standing or seated with a resistance band to build confidence.

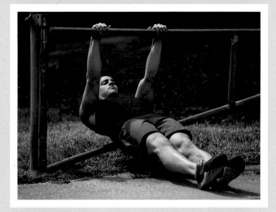

01 Lie on your back directly under the bar. Grasp the bar with an underhand grip (palms facing away) and with your hands shoulder width or closer.

CONTRACT ABS, KEEP BODY COMPLETELY STRAIGHT.

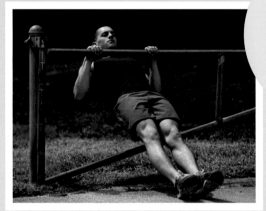

02 Pull yourself up until your chest touches the bar. Pause.

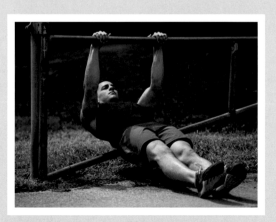

03 Lower yourself back down with control.

PIKE

The pike, or leg raise, is the one ab exercise we always come back to, because leg raises are a simple yet highly effective way to target the lower abs and hip flexors.

MORE DIFFICULT

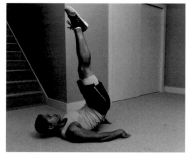

Modify range of motion: At the end of step 2, add a hip lift to increase ROM and work the lower abdominals and pelvic floor harder.

LESS DIFFICULT

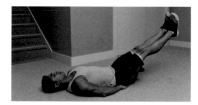

Modify range of motion: Decrease the workload by only partially lowering the legs in step 3. The less the legs drop, the easier.

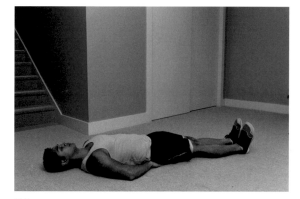

01 Lie on your back and place your hands, palms down, under your buttocks to help maintain a neutral pelvic position. Keep your legs as straight as possible and squeeze them together.

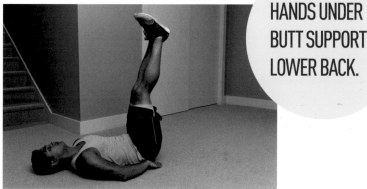

HANDS UNDER BUTT SUPPORT LOWER BACK.

02 Slowly raise your legs until they're perpendicular to the floor. Hold the contraction at the top for a second.

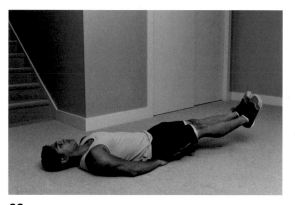

03 Slowly lower your feet to within 2.5cm (1in) of the floor. When performing reps, don't let the legs touch the floor.

INVERTED BODYWEIGHT ROW

This exercise balances the muscles used in press-ups and bench presses, helping with back strength and shoulder stability.

MORE DIFFICULT

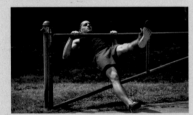

Modify stability and range of motion: Raise a foot to decrease stability and challenge trunk stabilization. Switch feet halfway through the reps.

LESS DIFFICULT

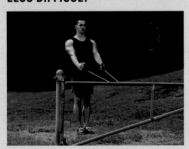

Modify stability and points of contact: Perform this exercise standing or seated with a resistance band to build confidence.

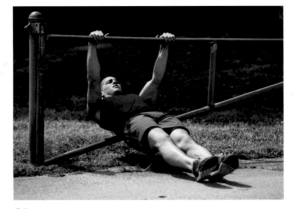

01 Lie on your back directly under the bar. Grab the bar with an overhand grip (palms facing away), and your hands wider than your shoulders.

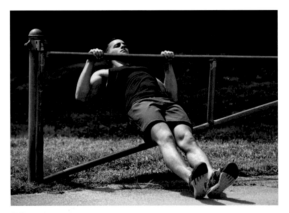

02 Pull yourself up until your chest touches the bar. Pause.

Keep your scapular retraction going during both the concentric and eccentric motions of the row. More specifically, try to pinch your shoulder blades together for the entire duration of the exercise.

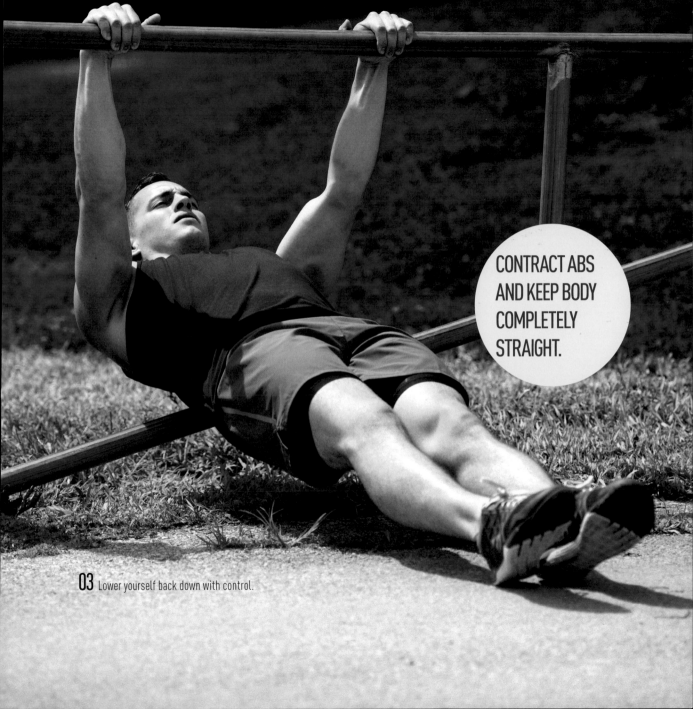

CONTRACT ABS AND KEEP BODY COMPLETELY STRAIGHT.

03 Lower yourself back down with control.

PULL-UP

Pull-ups are undoubtedly the best exercise for your upper back, and arguably one of the best exercises for the human body.

MORE DIFFICULT

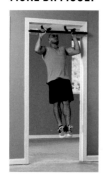

Modify speed: In step 3, slowly straighten your arms as you lower over a count of four to perform an eccentric muscle contraction that builds strength.

LESS DIFFICULT

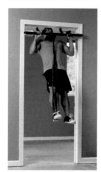

Modify points of contact and stability: For the entire exercise, use a band or place a foot on a chair to assist the pull-up by adding leverage.

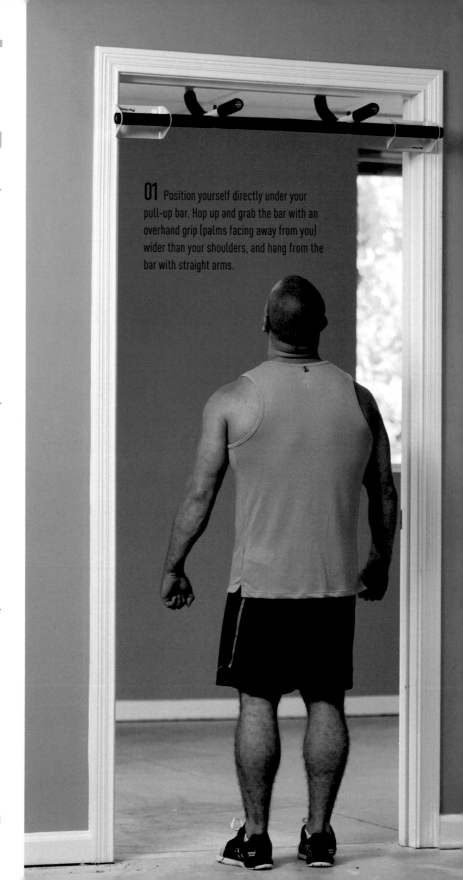

01 Position yourself directly under your pull-up bar. Hop up and grab the bar with an overhand grip (palms facing away from you) wider than your shoulders, and hang from the bar with straight arms.

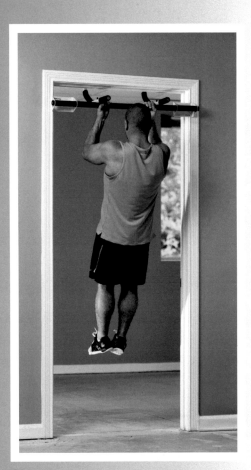

ISOLATE BACK
AND BICEPS.
DON'T SWING!

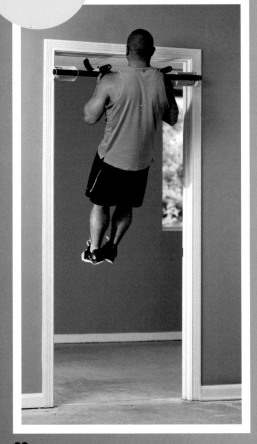

03 Lower yourself down with control. Repeat only steps 2
and 3 when performing reps.

The Guinness World record for
most pull-ups in one minute is 41
repetitions, performed by Ronald
Copper Jr, on 2 June, 2013.

02 Pull yourself up until your chin is above
the bar. Pause.

DOWN DOG PRESS-UP

Down dog press-ups are without question one of the best bodyweight exercises for your shoulders, allowing you to build the strength to perform gravity-defying wall walks and even handstand press-ups.

MORE DIFFICULT

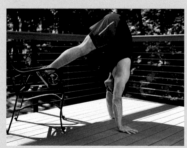

Modify body angle: During the entire exercise, elevate your feet on any available prop to decline the body and transfer a greater proportion of weight into the upper body

LESS DIFFICULT

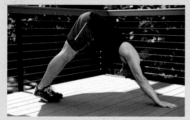

Modify body angle: In step 2, move your feet farther from your hands, so weight is more evenly distributed through the core.

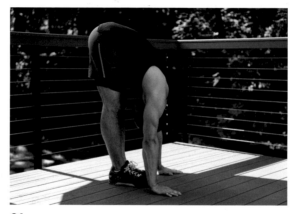

01 Begin by standing tall, then fold forwards from the hips until your hands are on the floor.

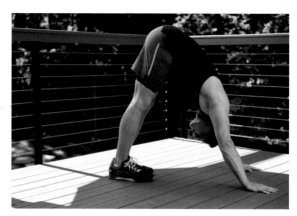

02 Walk your hands away from your body until you form a triangle with the ground. The farther your hands are from your feet, the easier the exercise becomes, because the muscles of the chest and back assist the shoulders. You're now in the down dog position; stay there for the remainder of the exercise.

> The shoulder is made up of three bones, as well as associated muscles, ligaments, and tendons. It's the most mobile joint in the human body.

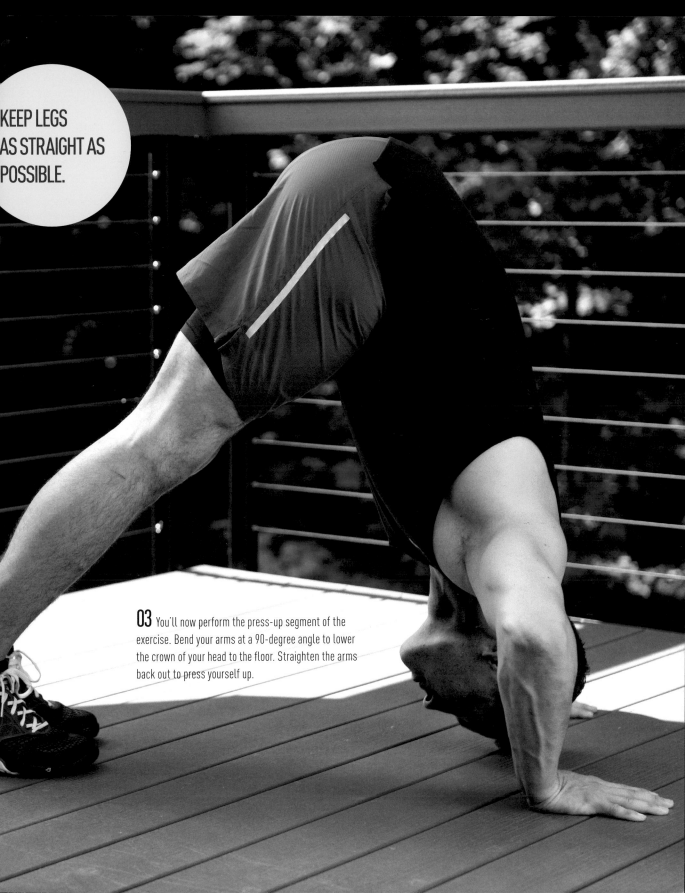

KEEP LEGS
AS STRAIGHT AS
POSSIBLE.

03 You'll now perform the press-up segment of the exercise. Bend your arms at a 90-degree angle to lower the crown of your head to the floor. Straighten the arms back out to press yourself up.

BURPEE

The Burpee is the undisputed bastion of the bodyweight revolution. Each rep incinerates calories and works virtually the entire body.

MORE DIFFICULT

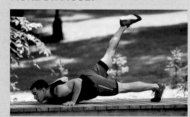

Modify points of contact: In step 3, elevate an arm, leg, or both to decrease stability and require greater core strength.

LESS DIFFICULT

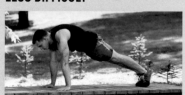

Modify range of motion: Remove the press-up in step 3 to perform squat thrusts, decreasing the work for the upper body.

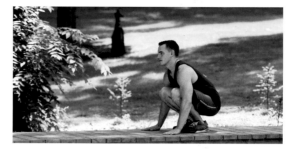

01 With your feet hip-width apart, bend your knees and bring your hands to the ground just in front of your feet.

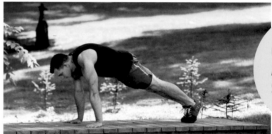

02 Hop your feet back into a plank position.

CONTRACT ABS, KEEP BODY STRAIGHT.

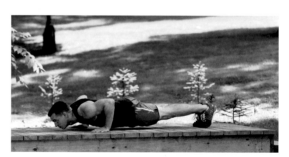

03 Perform one press-up with your core engaged.

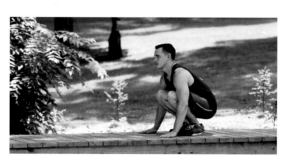

04 Jump to bring your feet back to your hands, shifting your weight into the heels and lifting your chest.

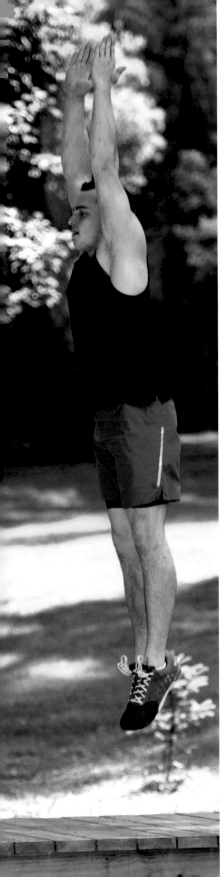

05 Jump upwards into the air with your arms extended straight above your head, palms facing each other. In mid-air, your arms, back, and legs should be straight and your toes should be pointed.

Try this ...

Vary Burpees by changing the hand position in the press-up portion of step 3. This engages other muscles of the chest, back, and arms, and forces you to compensate and balance in different ways.

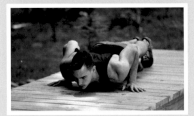

MILITARY PRESS-UP
Performing a military press-up isolates and engages the triceps.

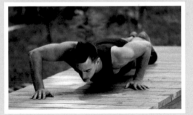

STAGGERED PRESS-UP
Decrease stability and help strengthen the serratus anterior with a staggered press-up.

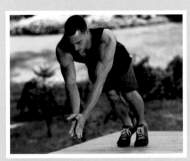

CLAP PRESS-UP
Use more power and build strength by performing a plyometric clap press-up.

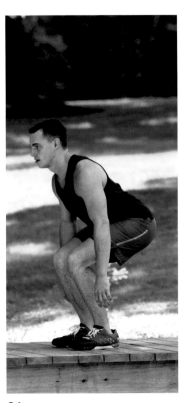

06 Land softly with a slight bend at your knees, hips, and ankles.

MILITARY PRESS-UP

Military press-ups change up hand position, exerting greater pressure on the triceps than a standard press-up. Narrowing the hand width decreases the base of support, challenging the core.

MORE DIFFICULT

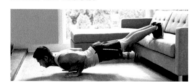

Modify body angle: In all steps, elevate your feet on a chair or box to decline the body and transfer weight into the upper body and core.

LESS DIFFICULT

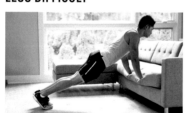

Modify body angle: In all steps, elevate your upper body (or kneel) to decrease the weight being moved by arms and shoulders.

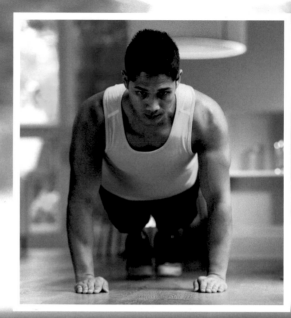

01 Assume a full plank or traditional press-up position, with the body balanced between the toes and hands. Position the hands directly under the shoulders, but not wider than the shoulders.

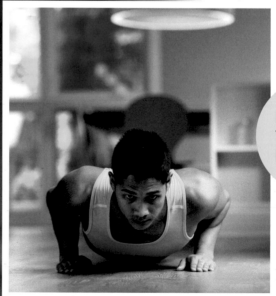

KEEP ELBOWS TIGHT AGAINST RIBCAGE.

02 Keeping the elbows and arms tight against your sides, bend your elbows and lower your body to the floor.

Due to the increased load on the triceps, military press-ups are difficult to execute with correct form. If you feel your hips lifting, either perform the press-ups on your knees, or revert to a standard press-up.

03 Once your elbows are slightly beyond 90 degrees, push up through your hands, straightening your arms to return to the starting position.

ELBOW BRIDGE

Elbow bridges are an excellent alternative to inverted bodyweight rows because they don't require a bar. This exercise engages the upper back and helps balance pushing exercises such as press-ups.

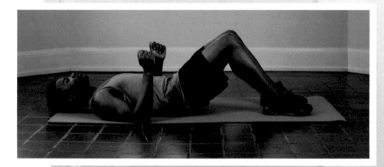

01 Lie on your back with your legs bent and the soles of your feet on the floor. Tuck your arms against your ribcage, with your elbows touching the floor.

MORE DIFFICULT

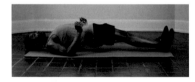

Modify points of contact and stability: Instead of bending the knees, keep legs straight in all steps, resting only your heels on the floor to increase demand on your core.

LESS DIFFICULT

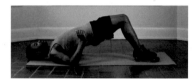

Modify speed: In step 2, hold for only three seconds to decrease the work-to-rest ratio.

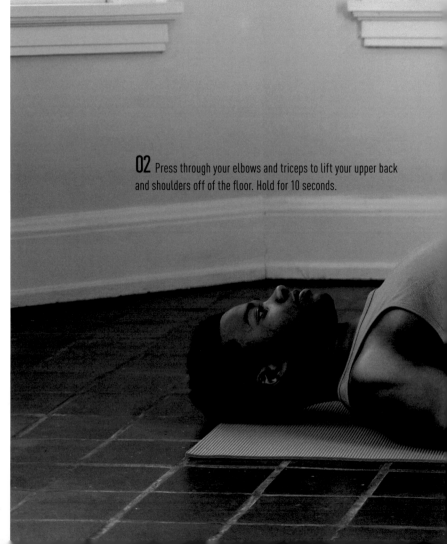

02 Press through your elbows and triceps to lift your upper back and shoulders off of the floor. Hold for 10 seconds.

Try to keep even pressure through your feet during this exercise. Make sure to connect the heel, and the pads of the big and little toes, with the ground.

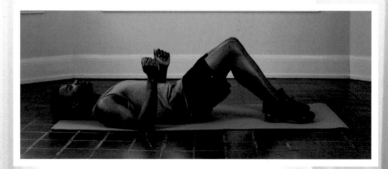

03 Lower yourself back down with control.

TUCK HIPS AND PELVIS SO SACRUM LIES FLAT.

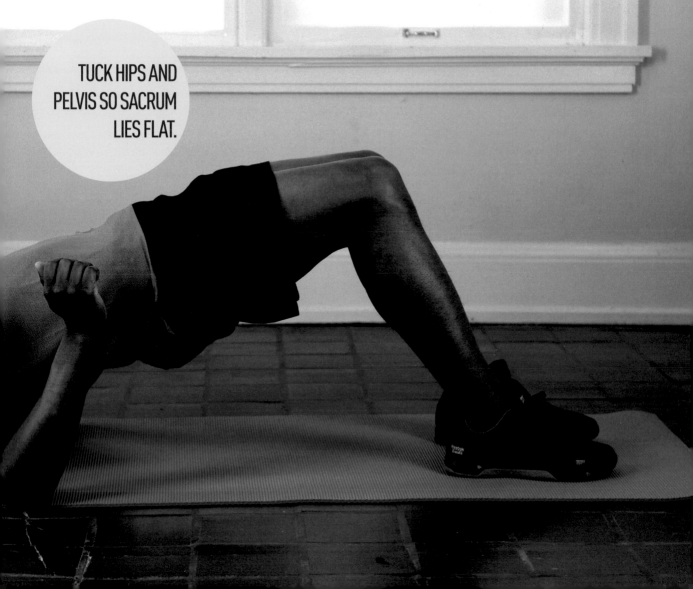

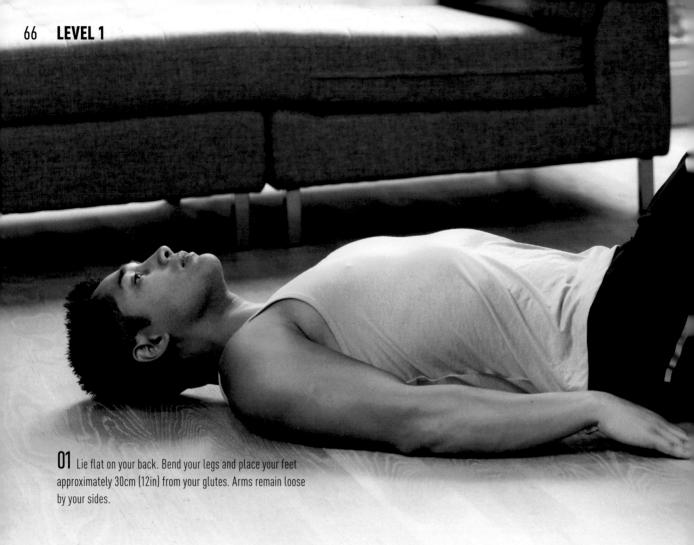

01 Lie flat on your back. Bend your legs and place your feet approximately 30cm (12in) from your glutes. Arms remain loose by your sides.

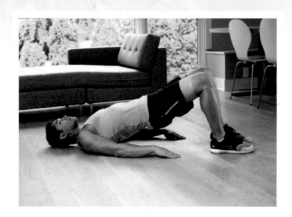

02 Pressing evenly through the soles of the feet, squeeze the glutes, and lift the hips until you form a straight line from shoulders to knees. Pause at the top of the motion and hold for 1–2 seconds.

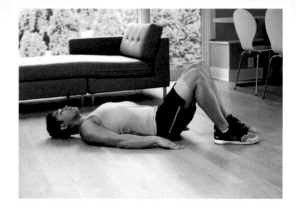

03 Lower back down to the floor under control.

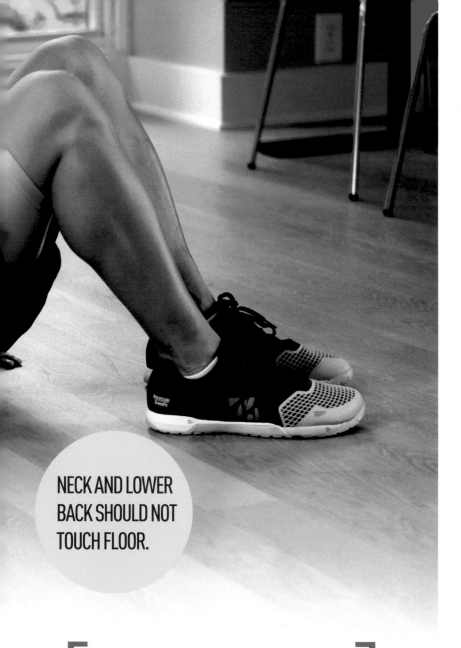

NECK AND LOWER BACK SHOULD NOT TOUCH FLOOR.

[
Try to distribute your weight evenly across both feet (heel, big toe, and little toe), squeeze the glutes, and avoid pushing out your ribcage as that will put pressure on your neck.
]

PELVIC PEEL

The pelvic peel strengthens the hips, hamstrings, and glutes while simultaneously stretching the quadriceps and hip flexors. Pelvic peels are excellent if you suffer from pelvic back pain because they work the muscles that support and stabilize the pelvis.

MORE DIFFICULT

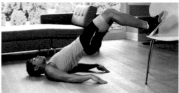

Modify body angle: For all steps, elevate your feet to decline the body and increase the height at which you have to lift your hips.

LESS DIFFICULT

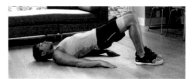

Modify speed: Instead of lifting and lowering, hold at the highest point in step 2 to create a strength-building isometric hold.

FORWARDS HINGE

The forwards hinge will help you gain awareness of the hips and correct use of the rear chain (hips, glutes, hamstrings). It may even help alleviate knee pain and increase the depth of your squats.

MORE DIFFICULT

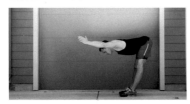

Modify range of motion and stability: Extend your arms in all steps. This lengthens your body, making your core work harder.

LESS DIFFICULT

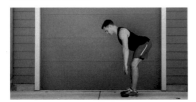

Modify range of motion: In step 2, decrease the angle of your hip hinge and slightly bend the knees, lessening the stress on the hamstrings.

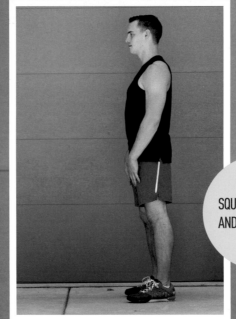

01 Stand with your feet shoulder-width apart and arms relaxed, with fingertips resting on the front of your thighs.

SQUEEZE GLUTES AND ENGAGE ABS.

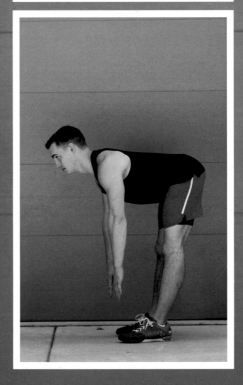

02 Hinge the hips back and fold forwards, keeping your back flat. Hold this position for 3–5 seconds.

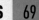

[
Push your hips back as far
as you can until you feel a
slight discomfort as you
stretch your hamstrings.
]

03 Return to the standing position.

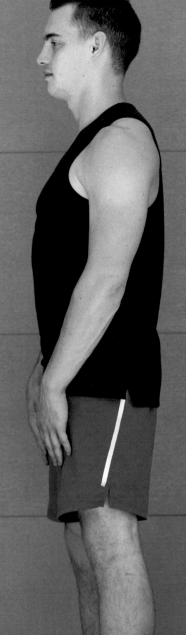

BACKWARDS BURPEE

The opposite of a classic Burpee, the backwards Burpee is performed facing upwards, which requires greater lower body activation than its better-known relative.

MORE DIFFICULT

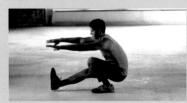

Modify stability: Perform on a single leg. This requires you to perform a muscle-building one-legged pistol squat to return to the starting position, which increases stability.

LESS DIFFICULT

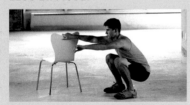

Modify stability: Place your hands on a chair or box when in standing position to help you perform with confidence and focus on form.

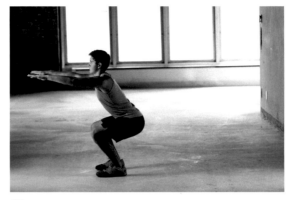

01 From a standing position, lower yourself to the floor and into a squat with your arms extended.

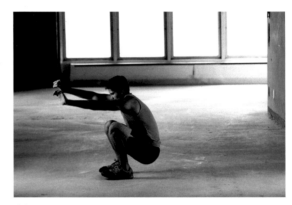

02 Round your back and engage your core as you lower your hips towards the floor.

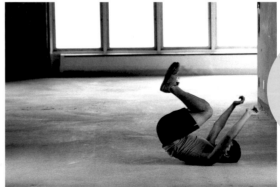

03 Starting from your thoracic spine, roll backwards through the lumbar spine with arms extended at sides for stability.

WHEN ROLLING, MAINTAIN A HOLLOW BODY POSITION WITH CORE ENGAGED.

A recent study shows that people who can sit or stand with little or no support from their hands or knees live the longest.

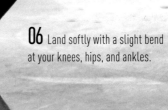

06 Land softly with a slight bend at your knees, hips, and ankles.

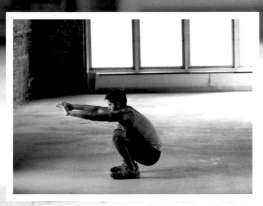

04 Roll forwards, reversing the motion from step 3 and ending with the weight in your heels, feet on the floor in a squat with arms extended for stability.

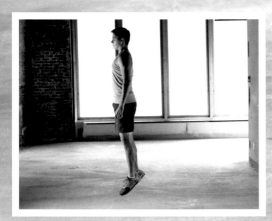

05 Jump up from the squat position.

X-JACK

This twist on the traditional jumping jack will boost your metabolism and tone your legs, core, shoulders, and back.

MORE DIFFICULT

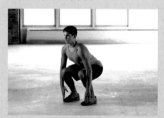

Modify speed: Hold the squat in step 1 for a count of four, creating a brief isometric hold and removing momentum.

LESS DIFFICULT

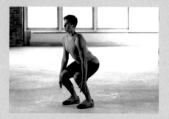

Modify range of motion: Decrease the squat depth in step 1 for a more cardiovascular exercise, replacing frequency for depth.

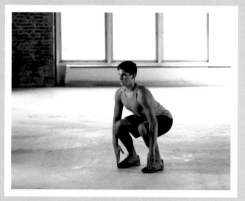

01 With feet shoulder-width apart, bend from your hips, knees, and ankles, and drop into a squat position. If you can, touch your toes with your fingertips.

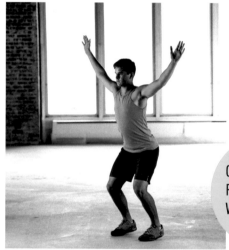

02 Jump out of the squat position. As you jump, straighten your legs and raise your arms overhead, crossing your wrists to make an X.

CHEST UP, LOOK FORWARDS, KEEP WEIGHT IN HEELS.

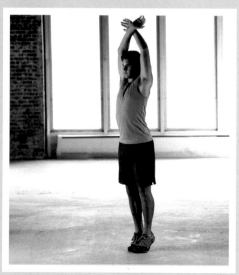

03 Land with your feet together, weight on balls of feet.

DIP

This targeted exercise isolates the triceps and strengthens the muscles surrounding the shoulder joint, providing protection and preventing injury.

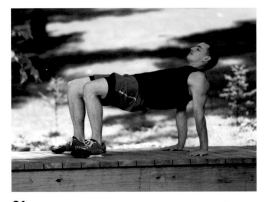

01 Sit with your feet flat on the floor in front of you and knees slightly bent. Lean back and place your hands on the floor behind your hips, fingers pointing towards your toes. Elevate the hips by engaging the core, hamstrings, and glutes.

MORE DIFFICULT

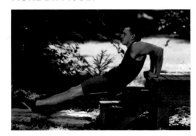

Modify range of motion: For all steps, elevate your hands on a prop and extend your legs to increase the workload on the core.

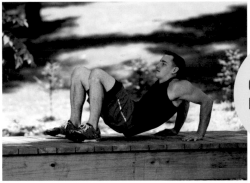

CHEST UP, LOOK FORWARDS.

02 Bend your elbows, lowering your buttocks until they're just above the ground.

LESS DIFFICULT

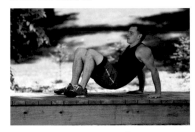

Modify body angle: In step 2, lower more shallowly, shifting weight from the upper body into the core and legs while you build strength.

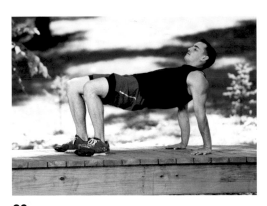

03 Straighten your arms and bring your hips back up to the starting position.

HANGING SCAPULA RETRACTION

This is a relatively basic exercise, but it's essential for shoulder and back health and will add gains to your bench press.

MORE DIFFICULT

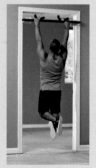

Modify speed: Instead of repeating steps 3 and 4, squeeze and hold the shoulder blades for the duration of the exercise. This creates a strength-building isometric hold.

LESS DIFFICULT

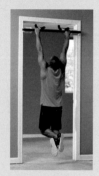

Modify speed: After step 2, omit the remaining steps. Instead, hang from the bar without shrugging the shoulders. This builds strength in the upper body and in your grip.

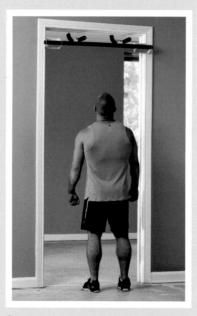

01 Position yourself directly under the pull-up bar.

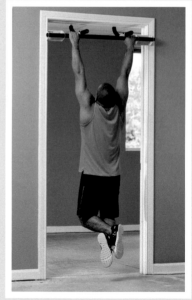

02 Hop up and grab the bar with an overhand grip wider than your shoulders, and settle into a dead hang position with shoulders pulled back and down (known as "packed").

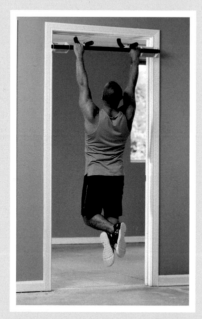

03 Lift your body by squeezing your shoulder blades together, and hold 3 seconds, with no bend in your arms. As you squeeze, your chest will decline and lower back will arch slightly.

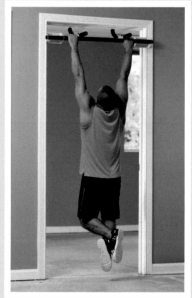

04 Slowly lower back to the dead hang position. Repeat steps 3 and 4 for the duration of the exercise.

BACK LUNGE

The back lunge is a simple, low-impact way to strengthen the quadriceps, hamstrings, gluteus maximus, and calves.

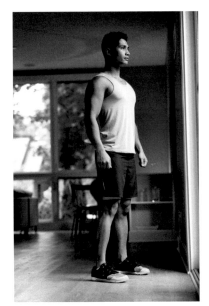

01 Stand tall with hands at your side.

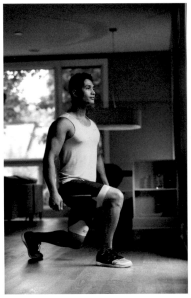

02 Take a large step back with your left foot. Lower hips so right thigh is parallel to the floor and right knee is directly over ankle. Left knee should be bent at a 90-degree angle.

MORE DIFFICULT

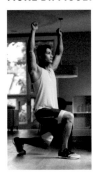

In all steps, extend arms overhead to decrease stability. This requires activation of the core to balance.

LESS DIFFICULT

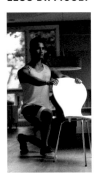

Modify stability: During the entire exercise, hold on to a chair or other prop to aid balance. This allows you to perform the exercise with greater confidence, and focus on the depth of the exercise.

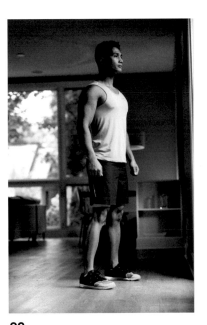

03 Return to a standing position by pressing through heel of right foot and bringing left foot forwards, standing tall to engage the core. Repeat, swapping legs.

CHEST UP, LOOK FORWARDS.

PRESS-UP JACK

Press-up jacks fuse cardiovascular jumping jacks with muscle-building press-ups for a killer compound exercise that torches calories.

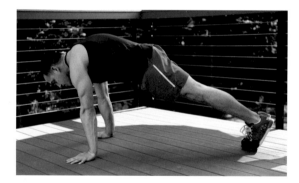

01 Assume a full plank or traditional press-up position with your body balanced between the toes and hands, with hands wider than shoulders and feet side by side.

MORE DIFFICULT

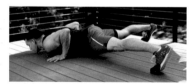

Modify points of contact: Change hand position to a military, diamond, or staggered press-up position to decrease leverage and stability.

LESS DIFFICULT

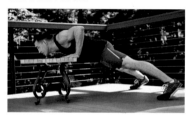

Modify body angle: During the entire exercise, use any available prop to elevate your upper body into an incline.

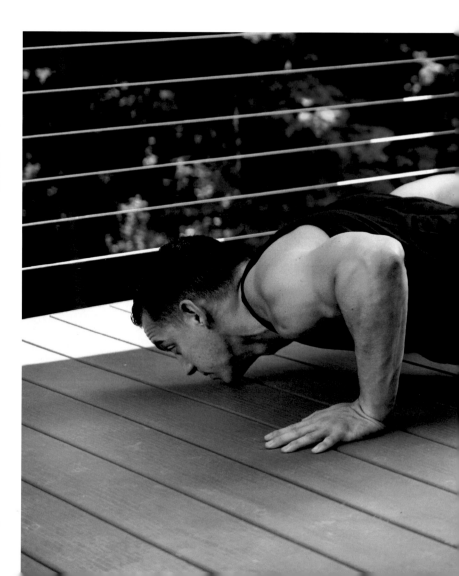

X marks the spot. Press-up jacks require incredible trunk stability and core strength and they will help you find some buried treasure – your six-pack abs.

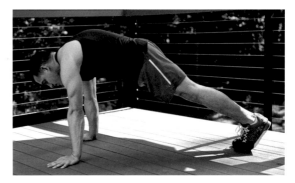

03 Press up through your hands, straightening the arms and hopping the feet closed to return to the starting position. Repeat steps 2 and 3 with controlled speed for the number of reps required.

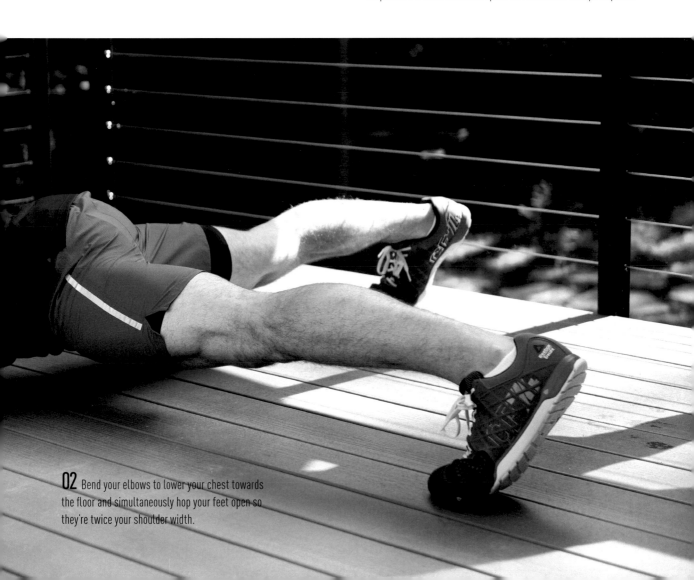

02 Bend your elbows to lower your chest towards the floor and simultaneously hop your feet open so they're twice your shoulder width.

BRIDGE KICK

Comprising part triceps dip, part pelvic peel, and part single-leg pike, this functional compound exercise requires you to activate the glutes to elevate the hips.

MORE DIFFICULT

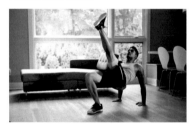

Modify range of motion and reps: In step 2, perform one full rep but lower only halfway instead of fully, then press back up to the highest point of the exercise for 1.5 reps.

LESS DIFFICULT

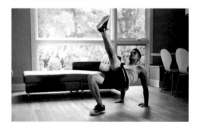

Modify speed: Hold the elevated kicking position in step 2 for the entire exercise to create a strength-building isometric hold.

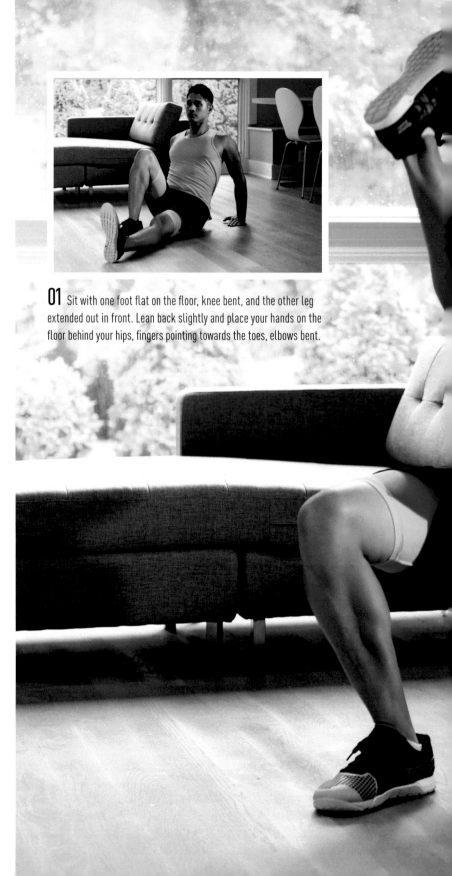

01 Sit with one foot flat on the floor, knee bent, and the other leg extended out in front. Lean back slightly and place your hands on the floor behind your hips, fingers pointing towards the toes, elbows bent.

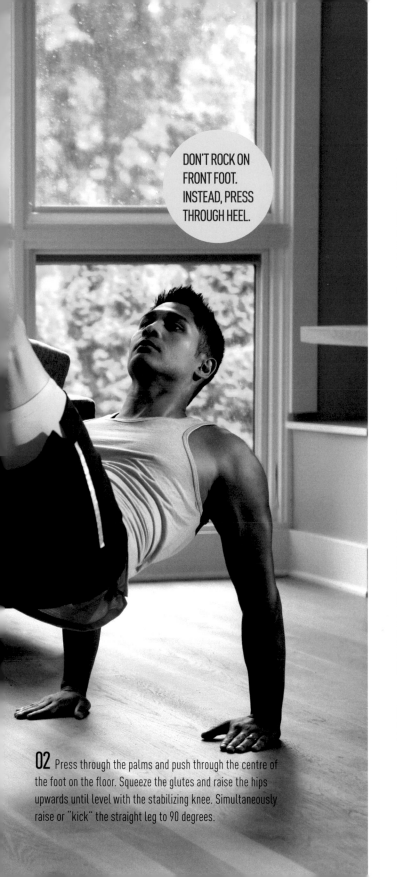

DON'T ROCK ON FRONT FOOT. INSTEAD, PRESS THROUGH HEEL.

[The glutes are one of the largest muscle groups in the body, so when you engage them you burn serious calories.]

02 Press through the palms and push through the centre of the foot on the floor. Squeeze the glutes and raise the hips upwards until level with the stabilizing knee. Simultaneously raise or "kick" the straight leg to 90 degrees.

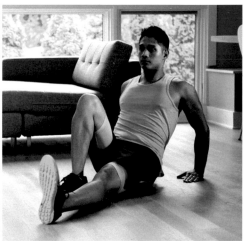

03 Bend your arms, bring your hips back to a slightly elevated starting position, and lower the extended leg back to the floor. Repeat steps 2 and 3 for the required number of reps.

WALL SIT

Wall sits make you hold a seated position – an isometric muscle contraction – so they strengthen the quadriceps and are a perfect exercise for people unaccustomed to squatting.

MORE DIFFICULT

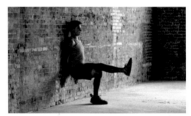

Modify points of contact: In all steps, hold a leg out in front to increase the workload for the supporting leg and challenge the core.

LESS DIFFICULT

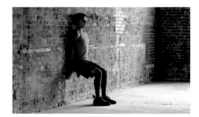

Modify body angle: In steps 2 and 3, slide down less, changing weight distribution and making it easier to sustain the sit.

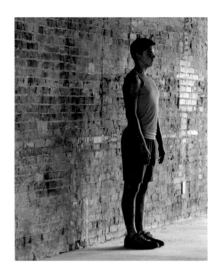

01 Stand approximately 45–60cm (18–24in) away from a wall.

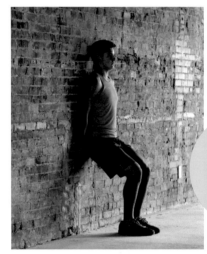

02 Lean back, pressing your torso against the wall.

ENGAGE CORE, PULL BELLY BUTTON IN TOWARDS SPINE.

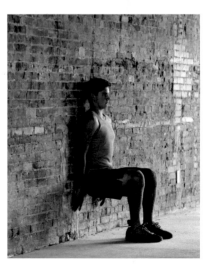

03 Slide down the wall until your thighs are parallel to the floor. The knees should be bent 90 degrees and straight above the ankles. Hold this position for the duration of the exercise.

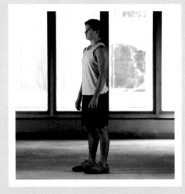

01 Stand tall, with your feet shoulder-width apart and toes pointing forwards.

SQUAT

This compound, full-body exercise primarily engages the thighs, hips, and buttocks. It also helps develop core strength by engaging the lower back and abdominals.

MORE DIFFICULT

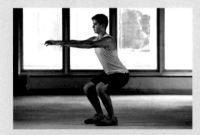

Modify range of motion and reps: In step 3, first perform a smaller half squat by standing halfway, then lower back into a full squat to perform 1.5 reps.

LESS DIFFICULT

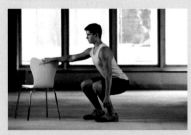

Modify stability: Hold a chair to provide balance and assistance as you build strength.

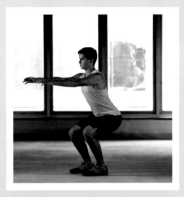

02 Inhale as you bend at the knee, lowering your body as if you're about to sit in a chair.

GLUTES TIGHT, PELVIS TUCKED, BELLY BUTTON IN.

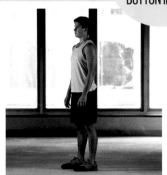

04 Exhale as you press through your heels, returning to the starting position. Squeeze your glutes as you stand, tucking your pelvis under and pulling the belly button inwards to engage your core. Repeat.

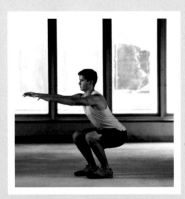

03 At the bottom of the movement, your knees should be at a 90-degree angle and your thighs parallel to the floor.

ARES WORKOUT

Tri-sets allow us to keep rest periods short while alternating between complementary exercises. The pyramid format (starting with a high number of reps and gradually reducing them with each round of a set of exercises) ensures focus on the quality of each rep. Ares translates to "battle" in ancient Greek, and Ares is the Greek god of war. This aptly named workout will help you build the back, shoulders, chest, and armoured core of a demi-god by combining push-and-pull bodyweight training classics.

Perform each set for five rounds, subtracting one rep per round where shown (pyramid format). Rest 30 seconds between rounds. Perform all sets and their exercises in order.

SET A

SQUAT	
10x	P081

STANDARD PRESS-UP	
5x, 4x, 3x, 2x, 1x	P048

PULL-UP	
5x, 4x, 3x, 2x, 1x	P056

🕐 REST 0:30 after each round of the set
🔄 REPEAT for five rounds in pyramid format

SET B

BACK LUNGE	
10x	P075

MILITARY PRESS-UP	
5x, 4x, 3x, 2x, 1x	P062

CHIN-UP	
5x, 4x, 3x, 2x, 1x	P050

🕐 REST 0:30 after each round of the set
🔄 REPEAT for five rounds in pyramid format

SET C

PELVIC PEEL	
10x	P066

DOWN DOG PRESS-UP	
5x, 4x, 3x, 2x, 1x	P058

INVERTED BODYWEIGHT ROW	
5x, 4x, 3x, 2x, 1x	P054

🕐 REST 0:30 after each round of the set
🔄 REPEAT for five rounds in pyramid format
🔄 **REPEAT sets A–C for a total of three rounds**

FINISHER
After three rounds of the sets, complete this finisher as fast as possible.

STANDARD PRESS-UP	
10x	P048

X-JACK	
20x	P072

BURPEE	
30x	P060

MOUNTAIN CLIMBER	
40x	P043

This is an AsFAP (As Fast As Possible) finisher. Remember: form first, speed second, but push as hard as you can to boost your metabolism and improve your calorie burn.

PERSEUS WORKOUT

This introduces the submax rep concept: performing a little less than your maximum number of reps. This focus on quality over quantity, and depth and ROM rather than reps, puts an emphasis on injury-free strength gains. In Greek mythology, Perseus was the first hero, and it will take a heroic effort to complete this total body workout.

Perform three full rounds with no rest between exercises or rounds.

SQUAT	
15x	P081
STANDARD PRESS-UP	
submax*	P048
BACK LUNGE	
12x each leg	P075
INVERTED BODYWEIGHT ROW	
submax*	P054
MILITARY PRESS-UP	
submax*	P062
DEAD HANG	
0:30	P042

↻ REPEAT for a total of three rounds

*Submax = 80 per cent of your max number of reps. If you're unsure of your max number of reps, perform the first round to failure (max) and subsequent rounds to 80 per cent of that max number – e.g., max = 10 reps, submax = 8 reps.

FINISHER

Perform the exercises in order, for the prescribed periods of time, including the rests.

SET A

STANDARD PRESS-UP	
0:20	P048
X-JACK	
0:20	P072
MOUNTAIN CLIMBER	
0:20	P043

🕐 REST 0:30

SET B

SQUAT	
0:20	P081
BACK LUNGE	
0:20	P075
ALTERNATING LATERAL LUNGE	
0:20	P046

🕐 REST 0:30

SET C

BURPEE	
0:20	P060
PRESS-UP JACK	
0:20	P076
BACKWARDS BURPEE	
0:20	P070

🕐 REST 0:30

↻ REPEAT sets A–C for a total of three rounds

ROUND THE WORLD

This workout is named after the circular motion of the first three exercises and the cyclical circuit-style repetition of the two sets. It will engage the large muscles of the lower body, forging a strong foundation while simultaneously supercharging the metabolism.

This may be a lower body-focussed workout, but keep your core engaged at all times by tightening the abdominals as if readying to take a blow to the body.

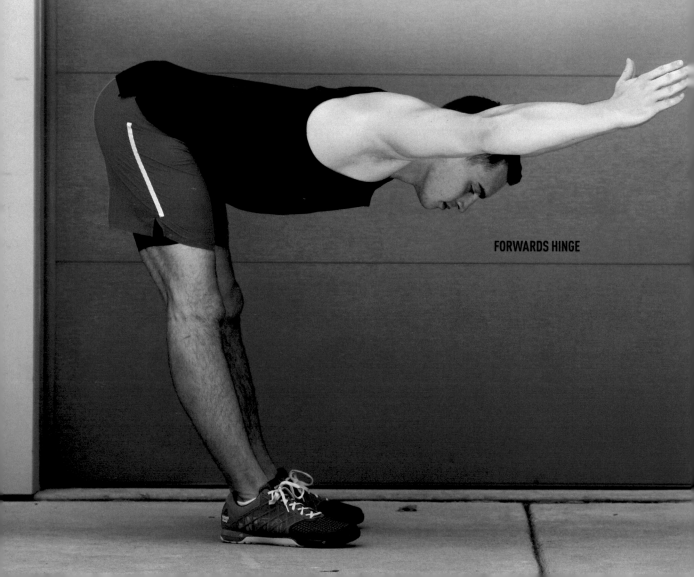

FORWARDS HINGE

Perform as many reps as you can of all exercises within the prescribed periods of time, and rest after each set.

 SET A

SQUAT

| 0:30 | **P**081 |

ALTERNATING LATERAL LUNGE

| 0:30 | **P**046 |

BACK LUNGE

| 0:30 | **P**075 |

WALL SIT

| 0:30 | **P**080 |

🕐 REST 0:30

SET B

PELVIC PEEL

| 0:30 | **P**066 |

BRIDGE KICK

| 0:30 each side | **P**078 |

FORWARDS HINGE

| 0:30 | **P**068 |

🕐 REST 0:30

↻ **REPEAT sets A–B for a total of three rounds**

PIKE

| 0:30 | **P**053 |

REVERSE PLANK BRIDGE

| 0:30 | **P**044 |

🕐 REST 0:30

↻ REPEAT Core Chaos for a total of six rounds

CORE CHAOS

After three rounds of the sets, complete these core exercises.

THOR WORKOUT

In Norse mythology, Thor is a hammer-wielding god associated with thunder, lightning bolts, oak trees, and, above all else, great strength! This total body workout isolates some of the largest muscles in the body, forging strong, lean muscle. It alternates high-rep exercises with exercises performed submaximally.

> If 15 reps is too high for each of the rowing exercises in this set, then perform these submaximally, but try to add a pause as you squeeze the shoulder blades on every rep.

FINISHER
This finisher includes short and frequent rest periods.

Perform this set with no rest between exercises or rounds.

X-JACK	
15x	**P072**

STANDARD PRESS-UP	
submax*	**P048**

CLOSE-GRIP INVERTED ROW	
15x	**P052**

MILITARY PRESS-UP	
submax*	**P062**

INVERTED BODYWEIGHT ROW	
15x	**P054**

DOWN DOG PRESS-UP	
submax*	**P058**

DEAD HANG	
0:30	**P042**

↻ REPEAT the set for a total of three rounds

*Submax = 80 per cent of your max number of reps. If you're unsure of your max number of reps, perform the first round to failure (max) and subsequent rounds to 80 per cent of that max number – e.g., max = 10 reps, submax = 8 reps.

X-JACK	
work 0:20, rest 0:10	**P072**

MOUNTAIN CLIMBER	
work 0:20, rest 0:10	**P043**

BURPEE	
work 0:20, rest 0:10	**P060**

↻ REPEAT the finisher for a total of six rounds

SUPER CIRCUIT
THE 300

King Leonidas led his army of 300 Spartans to the battle of Thermopylae to face an entire Persian army. No doubt it took great courage, strength, and determination to face such odds. Those same credentials are required for this first super circuit. With the equivalent of 300 reps of Level 1's greatest exercises, this workout will test both your strength and stamina.

> When performing the Burpees and mountain climbers, aim to do at least the number of reps of the current round within the 30-second time frame.

In the list below, "R" means "round." Perform the exercises in each round in order, followed by a two-minute rest.

If you choose to undertake the bonus round, each single rep should be performed as slowly as you possibly can; aim for it to take 10 seconds to perform that one rep – five seconds up and five seconds down.

PULL-UP

R1 15x, R2 10x, R3 5x, Bonus 1x	P056

PELVIC PEEL

R1 15x, R2 10x, R3 5x, Bonus 1x	P066

STANDARD PRESS-UP

R1 15x, R2 10x, R3 5x, Bonus 1x	P048

BURPEE

0:30 all rounds	P060

PIKE

R1 15x, R2 10x, R3 5x, Bonus 1x	P053

SQUAT

R1 15x, R2 10x, R3 5x, Bonus 1x	P081

DOWN DOG PRESS-UP

R1 15x, R2 10x, R3 5x, Bonus 1x	P058

MOUNTAIN CLIMBER

0:30 all rounds	P043

INVERTED BODYWEIGHT ROW

R1 15x, R2 10x, R3 5x, Bonus 1x	P054

CHIN-UP

R1 15x, R2 10x, R3 5x, Bonus 1x	P050

🕐 REST 2:00 after each round

🔁 REPEAT for a total of three rounds, plus one bonus round if desired

SUPER CIRCUIT FIVE

Infamously known simply as "Five" in my gym, this three-set super circuit requires high output and high repetitions for a total of five rounds. Working a higher number of reps for this super set will help build your endurance and athletic performance, and will induce muscular hypertrophy (an increase in the size of skeletal muscle).

> During any timed exercise, aim for maximum capacity and work until absolute failure. For rep-based exercises, focus on controlled range of motion.

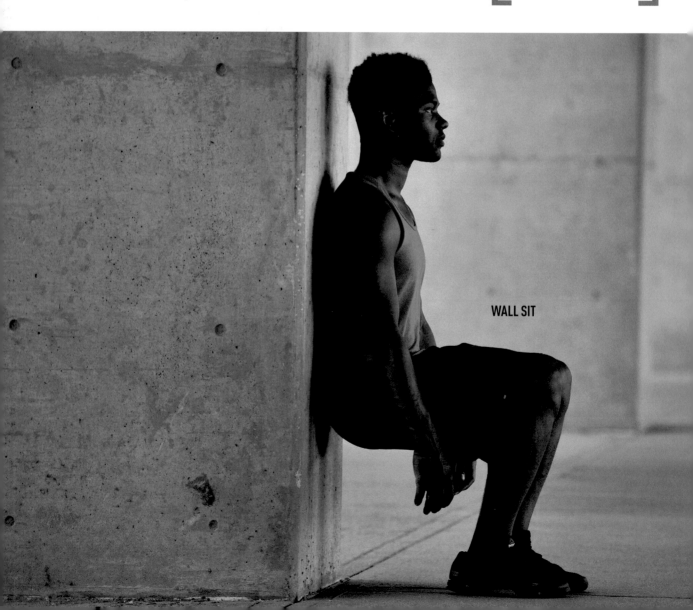

WALL SIT

Super Circuit Five can be performed in two different ways:
1. Perform each set for five rounds with a one-minute rest after each round, then move on to the next set.
2. Perform A, B, and C in order with a one-minute rest between each set and repeat in sequence for five rounds.

STANDARD PRESS-UP

20x	P048

DIP

20x	P073

WALL SIT

0:45	P080

PIKE

20x	P053

🕐 REST 1:00

REVERSE PLANK BRIDGE

0:45	P044

MILITARY PRESS-UP

20x	P062

SQUAT

20x	P081

CHIN-UP

10x	P050

🕐 REST 1:00

MOUNTAIN CLIMBER

0:45	P043

X-JACK

20x	P072

BACK LUNGE

20x each leg	P075

PULL-UP

10x	P056

🕐 REST 1:00

🔄 **REPEAT for a total of five rounds, either one set at a time or repeating sets in a sequence**

10 TO 1

This workout decreases from ten reps per round to just one. Squats, pull-ups, and dips, when combined in one workout, work almost every muscle in your body, including some of the largest.

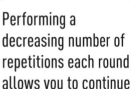

Performing a decreasing number of repetitions each round allows you to continue working and focussing on quality even when fatigued.

CORE KILLER
Perform all exercises in order for a total of six rounds with a one-minute rest halfway through and at the end. Total exercise time: eight minutes.

Perform the exercises in order – e.g., 10 squats, 10 pull-ups, 10 dips – then repeat the set for a total of ten rounds, subtracting one rep per round (pyramid format). No rest between rounds.

SQUAT

10x, 9x, 8x, 7x, 6x, 5x, 4x, 3x, 2x, 1x	P081

PULL-UP

10x, 9x, 8x, 7x, 6x, 5x, 4x, 3x, 2x, 1x	P056

DIP

10x, 9x, 8x, 7x, 6x, 5x, 4x, 3x, 2x, 1x	P073

↻ REPEAT for ten rounds in pyramid format

PIKE

0:20	P053

MOUNTAIN CLIMBER

0:20	P043

REVERSE PLANK BRIDGE

0:20	P044

↻ REPEAT Core Killer for three rounds
🕐 REST 1:00
↻ REPEAT Core Killer for three more rounds
🕐 REST 1:00

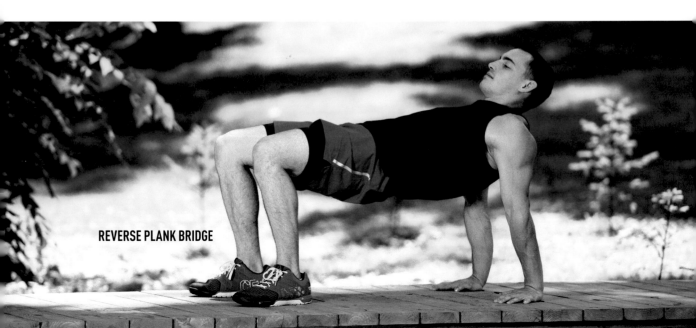

REVERSE PLANK BRIDGE

PUSH V PULL

Concentric versus eccentric muscle contractions; chest versus back; the anterior muscles of the body versus those on the posterior side – Push v Pull is the body's very own battle of the heavyweight champions. This workout utilizes the pyramid format of decreasing reps per round, which you'll do twice. Can you make it go the distance?

> Attempt to perform the rounds that have single reps of each exercise as slowly as possible.

CORE CHAOS
To finish, complete six full rounds of these core exercises. Total exercise time: nine minutes.

Perform the exercises in order – e.g., 5 standard press-ups, 5 pull-ups, 5 military press-ups, etc – then repeat the set for five rounds, subtracting one rep per round (pyramid format). Rest two minutes and perform five more rounds.

STANDARD PRESS-UP

5x, 4x, 3x, 2x, 1x	P048

PULL-UP

5x, 4x, 3x, 2x, 1x	P056

MILITARY PRESS-UP

5x, 4x, 3x, 2x, 1x	P062

INVERTED BODYWEIGHT ROW

5x, 4x, 3x, 2x, 1x	P054

DOWN DOG PRESS-UP

5x, 4x, 3x, 2x, 1x	P058

CHIN-UP

5x, 4x, 3x, 2x, 1x	P050

PRESS-UP JACK

5x, 4x, 3x, 2x, 1x	P076

CLOSE-GRIP INVERTED ROW

5x, 4x, 3x, 2x, 1x	P052

↻ REPEAT for five rounds in pyramid format
🕐 REST 2:00
↻ REPEAT for five more rounds in pyramid format

PIKE

0:30	P053

REVERSE PLANK BRIDGE

0:30	P044

🕐 REST 0:30
↻ REPEAT Core Chaos for a total of six rounds

DYNAMIC DUOS

A couplet is a pairing of two functional movements. The two should complement each other in the sense that one is a pull movement and the other a push movement. The benefit of couplets is that by offsetting a push movement with a pull movement, you give yourself time to "rest" while you're actively working, which decreases your down time and makes the workout more effective.

> If you begin to fatigue on the chin-ups, jump up to the bar, using momentum to help lift you, and slowly control your descent over a count of four. This eccentric contraction helps build strength.

CORE KILLER
Perform all exercises in order for a total of six rounds with a one-minute rest halfway through and at the end. Total exercise time: eight minutes.

Perform the sets as couplets – e.g., 10 dips followed by 10 chin-ups. Don't rest, but move immediately to eight reps of each exercise (decreasing the reps per round in a pyramid format). Complete all five rounds of a set before resting one minute and moving on to the next set.

 SET A

DIP	
10x, 8x, 6x, 4x, 2x	P073

CHIN-UP	
10x, 8x, 6x, 4x, 2x	P050

↻ REPEAT for five rounds in pyramid format
🕐 REST 1:00 before set B

 SET B

SQUAT	
10x, 8x, 6x, 4x, 2x	P081

INVERTED BODYWEIGHT ROW	
10x, 8x, 6x, 4x, 2x	P054

↻ REPEAT for five rounds in pyramid format
🕐 REST 1:00 before set C

 SET C

DOWN DOG PRESS-UP	
10x, 8x, 6x, 4x, 2x	P058

PELVIC PEEL	
10x, 8x, 6x, 4x, 2x	P066

↻ REPEAT for five rounds in pyramid format
🕐 REST 1:00

PIKE	
0:20	P053

MOUNTAIN CLIMBER	
0:20	P042

REVERSE PLANK BRIDGE	
0:20	P044

↻ REPEAT Core Killer for three rounds
🕐 REST 1:00
↻ REPEAT Core Killer for three more rounds
🕐 REST 1:00

HI-LO

Triplets, as the name suggests, combine three functional exercises, often complementary push and pull exercises. For Hi-Lo, the third item in each triplet is a dynamic high-intensity exercise to boost metabolism, and also to improve endurance and athletic performance.

[
If you're having a hard time recovering between sets, increase the rest period to two minutes.
]

Perform the sets as triplets – e.g., 10 press-ups, 10 hanging scapula retractions, and 45 seconds of mountain climbers. Don't rest, but move immediately to eight reps of each exercise in a pyramid format. Complete all five rounds of a set before resting one minute and moving on to the next set.

 SET A

STANDARD PRESS-UP	
10x, 8x, 6x, 4x, 2x	**P**048
HANGING SCAPULA RETRACTION	
10x, 8x, 6x, 4x, 2x	**P**074
MOUNTAIN CLIMBER	
0:45	**P**043

↻ REPEAT for five rounds in pyramid format
🕐 REST 1:00 before set B

SET B

SQUAT	
10x, 8x, 6x, 4x, 2x	**P**081
PELVIC PEEL	
10x, 8x, 6x, 4x, 2x	**P**066
X-JACK	
0:45	**P**072

↻ REPEAT for five rounds in pyramid format
🕐 REST 1:00 before set C

SET C

DIP	
10x, 8x, 6x, 4x, 2x	**P**073
INVERTED BODYWEIGHT ROW	
10x, 8x, 6x, 4x, 2x	**P**054
PRESS-UP JACK	
0:45	**P**076

↻ REPEAT for five rounds in pyramid format
🕐 REST 1:00 before set D

SET D

BACK LUNGE	
10x, 8x, 6x, 4x, 2x	**P**075
CHIN-UP	
10x, 8x, 6x, 4x, 2x	**P**050
BURPEE	
0:45	**P**060

↻ REPEAT for five rounds in pyramid format
🕐 REST 1:00

BURN

Based on intervals of 20 seconds of all-out exercise followed by 10 seconds of rest, Tabata training workouts incinerate body fat. Performing as many reps as you possibly can in 20 seconds will make your heart rate skyrocket. The high energy output allows you to tap the post-workout benefits of Tabata and high intensity interval training, which allows you to burn calories for up to 48 hours after the workout.

Always remember: form first, speed second. Push for maximum reps but not at the cost of your form, as this may lead to injury.

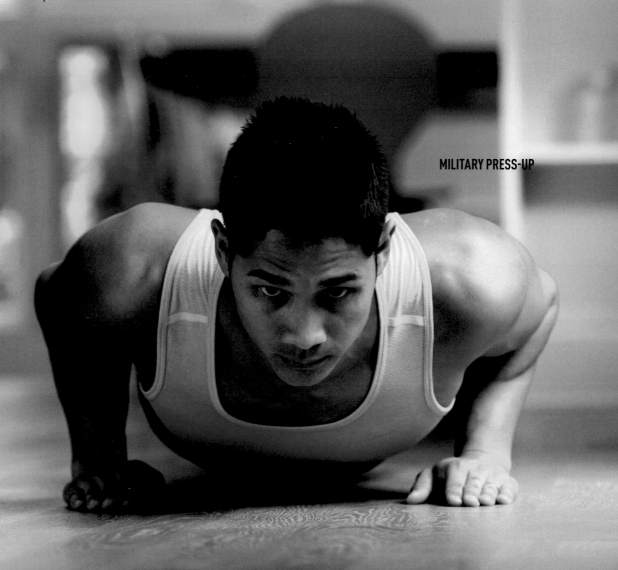

MILITARY PRESS-UP

Perform both exercises in each set three times. Rest one minute between each set. Total time for the workout should be 28 minutes.

 SET A

PRESS-UP JACK
| work 0:20, rest 0:10 | **P**076 |

BACKWARDS BURPEE
| work 0:20, rest 0:10 | **P**070 |

↻ REPEAT for three rounds
🕐 REST 1:00 before set B

 SET B

CHIN-UP
| work 0:20, rest 0:10 | **P**050 |

STANDARD PRESS-UP
| work 0:20, rest 0:10 | **P**048 |

↻ REPEAT for three rounds
🕐 REST 1:00 before set C

 SET C

BURPEE
| work 0:20, rest 0:10 | **P**060 |

CLOSE-GRIP INVERTED ROW
| work 0:20, rest 0:10 | **P**052 |

↻ REPEAT for three rounds
🕐 REST 1:00 before set D

SET D

PULL-UP
| work 0:20, rest 0:10 | **P**056 |

MILITARY PRESS-UP
| work 0:20, rest 0:10 | **P**062 |

↻ REPEAT for three rounds
🕐 REST 1:00 before set E

SET E

BACK LUNGE
| work 0:20, rest 0:10 | **P**075 |

MOUNTAIN CLIMBER
| work 0:20, rest 0:10 | **P**043 |

↻ REPEAT for three rounds
🕐 REST 1:00 before set F

SET F

PELVIC PEEL
| work 0:20, rest 0:10 | **P**066 |

DOWN DOG PRESS-UP
| work 0:20, rest 0:10 | **P**058 |

↻ REPEAT for three rounds
🕐 REST 1:00 before set G

SET G

DIP
| work 0:20, rest 0:10 | **P**073 |

INVERTED BODYWEIGHT ROW
| work 0:20, rest 0:10 | **P**054 |

↻ REPEAT for three rounds
🕐 REST 1:00

LEG DAY

A strong lower body means strong performance. Think about it: If you want to change direction in football or rugby, where does that move originate? It may be controlled by the core, but it's performed by the lower body accelerating and decelerating. The lower body also contains some of the largest muscles, so not only will you build a strong and solid foundation with this workout, but you'll also burn more calories than almost any other muscle group. In short, never skip leg day!

For more of a challenge, combine sets A and B into one eight-exercise workout and complete four rounds, eliminating the rest between sets to decrease your recovery time.

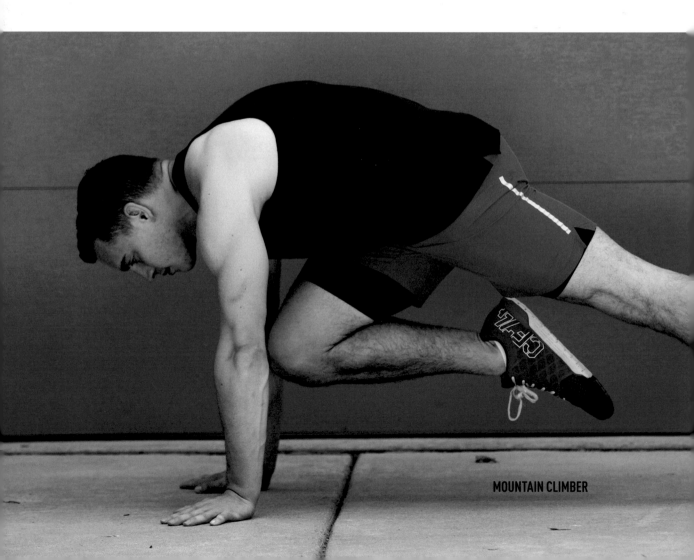

MOUNTAIN CLIMBER

Perform the exercises in order – e.g., 15 squats, 15 pelvic peels, 15 back lunges per leg, 30 seconds of reverse plank bridge. Don't rest, but move immediately to 10 reps of each exercise (pyramid format). Complete all four rounds of set A before resting two minutes and moving on to set B.

SET A

SQUAT

15x, 10x, 5x, 10x   P081

PELVIC PEEL

15x, 10x, 5x, 10x   P066

BACK LUNGE

15x each leg   P075

REVERSE PLANK BRIDGE

0:30   P044

↻ REPEAT for four rounds in pyramid format
🕐 REST 2:00 before set B

SET B

ALTERNATING LATERAL LUNGE

15x each leg   P046

FORWARDS HINGE

15x, 10x, 5x, 10x   P068

WALL SIT

0:30   P080

DEAD HANG

0:30   P042

↻ REPEAT for four rounds in pyramid format
🕐 REST 2:00

X-JACK

work 0:20, rest 0:10   P072

MOUNTAIN CLIMBER

work 0:20, rest 0:10   P043

BURPEE

work 0:20, rest 0:10   P060

↻ REPEAT the finisher for a total of six rounds

FINISHER
Perform six rounds.
Total time for finisher:
nine minutes.

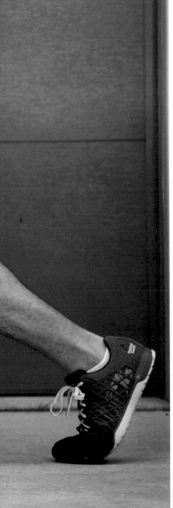

PROGRAMME

Programmes are structured so weeks 1 and 3 are the same, as are weeks 2 and 4. Work six days on and one off. Ideally you would structure it Monday to Saturday and rest Sunday, but if your schedule prevents this, or you need a midweek rest at first due to muscle soreness, schedule your rest day accordingly. Avoid switching the workouts within the programme, as this may adversely affect your rest time for a specific muscle group.

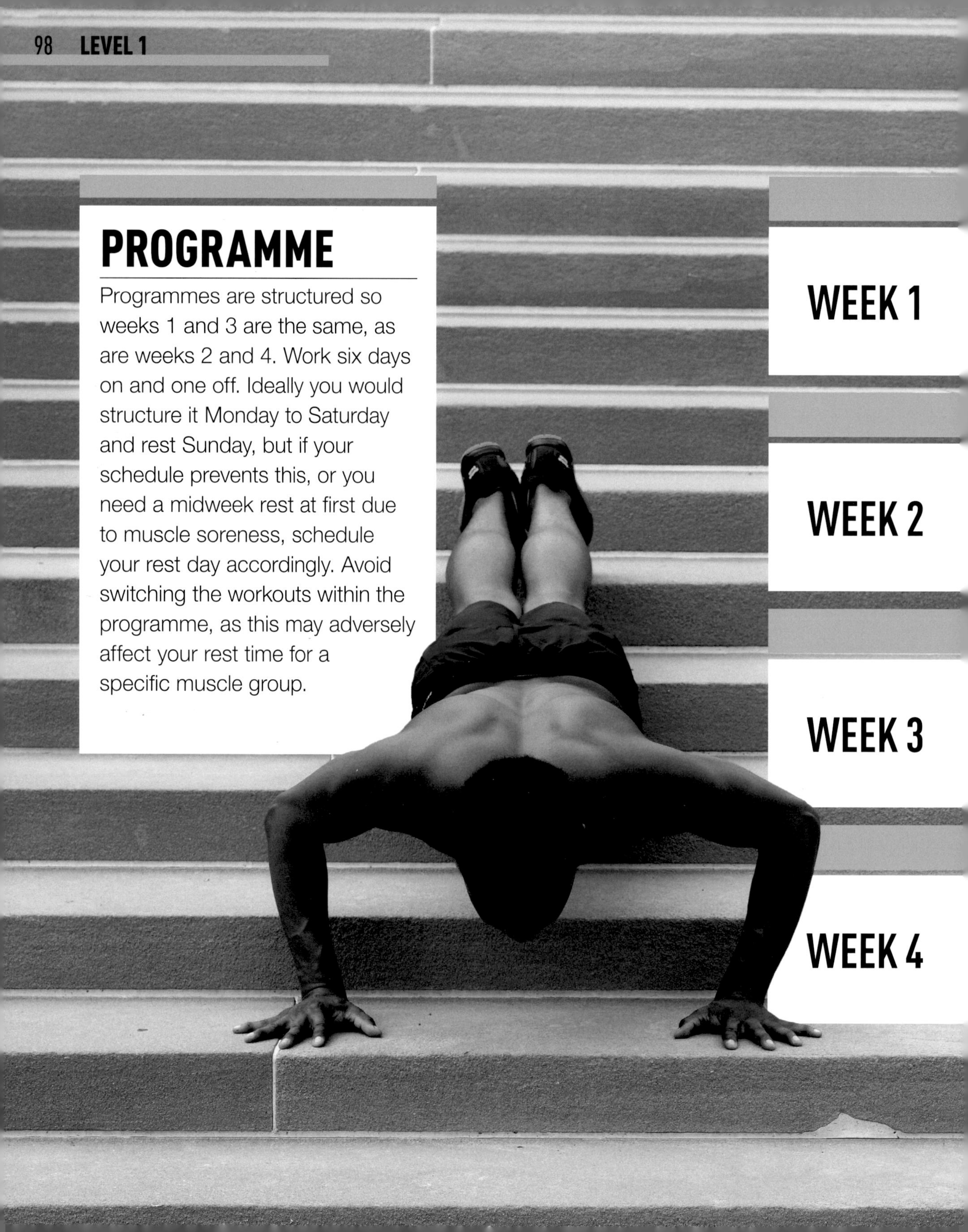

WEEK 1

WEEK 2

WEEK 3

WEEK 4

DAY **01**	DAY **02**	DAY **03**	DAY **04**	DAY **05**	DAY **06**
• ARES WORKOUT • FINISHER	• ROUND THE WORLD • CORE CHAOS	• PERSEUS WORKOUT • FINISHER	• 10 TO 1 • CORE KILLER	• THOR WORKOUT • FINISHER	• SUPER CIRCUIT THE 300

DAY **08**	DAY **09**	DAY **10**	DAY **11**	DAY **12**	DAY **13**
• LEG DAY • FINISHER	• PUSH V PULL • CORE CHAOS	• BURN	• DYNAMIC DUOS • CORE KILLER	• HI-LO	• SUPER CIRCUIT FIVE

DAY **15**	DAY **16**	DAY **17**	DAY **18**	DAY **19**	DAY **20**
• ARES WORKOUT • FINISHER	• ROUND THE WORLD • CORE CHAOS	• PERSEUS WORKOUT • FINISHER	• 10 TO 1 • CORE KILLER	• THOR WORKOUT • FINISHER	• SUPER CIRCUIT THE 300

DAY **22**	DAY **23**	DAY **24**	DAY **25**	DAY **26**	DAY **27**
• LEG DAY • FINISHER	• PUSH V PULL • CORE CHAOS	• BURN	• DYNAMIC DUOS • CORE KILLER	• HI-LO	• SUPER CIRCUIT FIVE

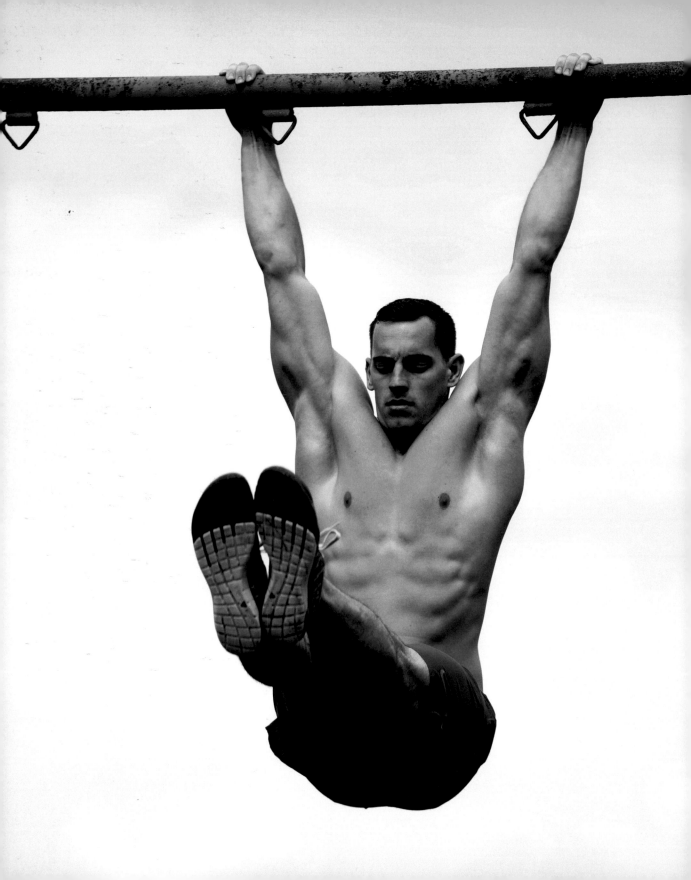

LEVEL 2

Level 2 builds upon the foundation and strength you developed in Level 1 and increases the challenge through multiplanar (more than one plane of motion) and dynamic stability (motion or rotation) exercises.

DEEP SQUAT

A full-body exercise, the deep squat primarily engages the quads, hips, and glutes. Dropping into a deep seated position requires greater hip mobility and flexibility than for a regular squat.

MORE DIFFICULT

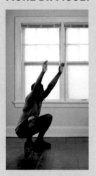

Modify stability: As you perform the entire exercise, extend your arms overhead to lengthen the torso, challenge your balance, and increase the work for the glutes and core.

LESS DIFFICULT

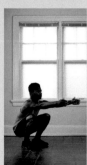

Modify stability: In step 2, extend your arms in front of your body to provide counterbalance.

DON'T LET KNEES BUCKLE INWARDS WHILE LOWERING.

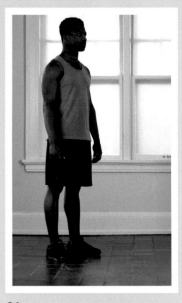

01 Stand tall with your feet shoulder-width apart and toes pointing forwards.

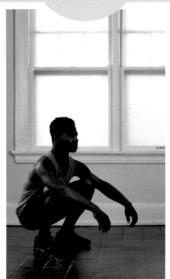

02 Inhale as you bend at the knee and lower your body until shins and thighs form an angle less than 90 degrees. Lower the hips until glutes touch calves and heels, or as far as possible.

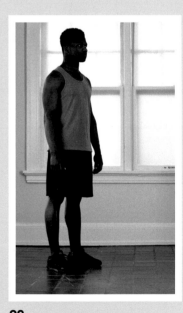

03 Pause, exhale, and press through your heels, returning to the starting position while squeezing your glutes, tucking your pelvis, and pulling the belly button in. Repeat steps 2 and 3 as prescribed.

SPIDERMAN PRESS-UP

Inspired by the agile superhero of the same name, this press-up will increase hip mobility, flexibility, and core strength.

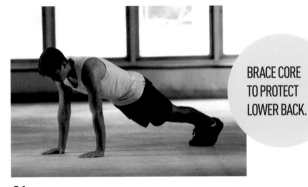

BRACE CORE TO PROTECT LOWER BACK.

01 Assume a standard press-up position, with palms just wider than shoulders, arms straight, and body in a rigid line, with weight balanced between arms and toes.

MORE DIFFICULT

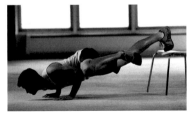

Modify body angle: Elevate your feet on a prop to decline the body and transfer more weight to the upper body.

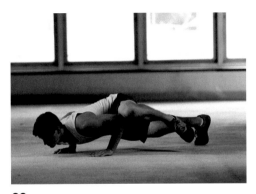

02 Bend your arms, bringing the chest down as you lift your left foot off of the floor. Rotate the left leg out to the side and pull your right knee up to your shoulder.

LESS DIFFICULT

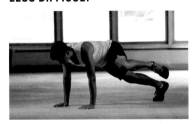

Modify stability: Instead of performing a press-up in steps 2 and 3, hold the plank position and roll the knee to the shoulder.

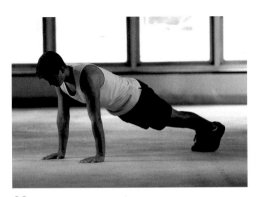

03 Bring your right foot back to the floor and push your body back up to the starting position. Repeat steps 2 and 3, alternating legs.

FRONT LUNGE

The front lunge is a simple, low-impact way to strengthen the quads, hamstrings, glutes, and calves.

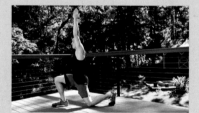

Modify stability: For the entire exercise, raise your hands overhead to challenge stability.

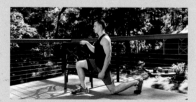

Modify stability: Hold on to any available prop to aid balance.

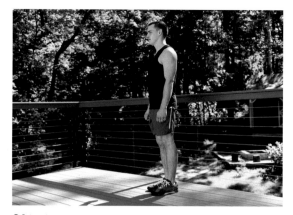

01 Stand straight, with arms at your side and core engaged.

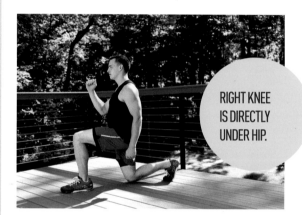

RIGHT KNEE IS DIRECTLY UNDER HIP.

02 Step your left foot forwards. Bending your right knee 90 degrees, lower your hips to bring your left thigh parallel to the floor and your left knee directly over your ankle.

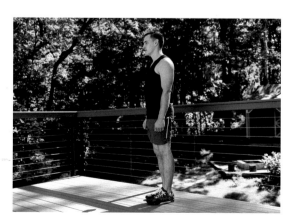

03 Return to standing by pressing through the heel of the left foot and bringing the foot backwards, standing tall to engage the core.

According to the American Council on Exercise, lunges are one of the most effective lower-body exercises. Studies prove strengthening the lower body can speed up metabolism and aid fat loss.

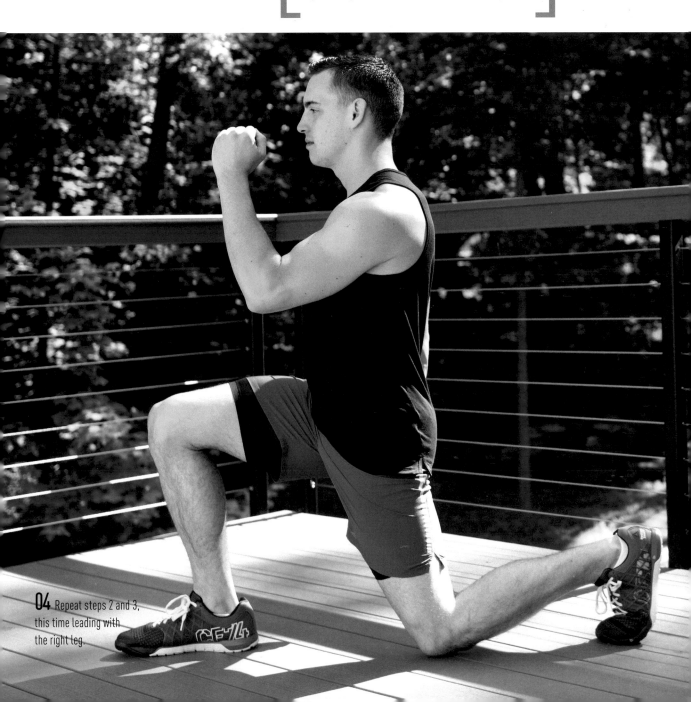

04 Repeat steps 2 and 3, this time leading with the right leg.

ALTERNATING CROSS-OVER LUNGE

Apart from building strength in the quads and glutes, this lunge also enhances balance, coordination, and agility.

MORE DIFFICULT

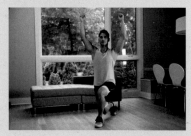

Modify stability: In all steps, hold arms overhead to decrease balance and add load to hips, glutes, and core.

LESS DIFFICULT

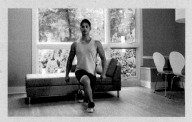

Modify stability: Instead of taking step 4, perform all repetitions to one side to increase stability by making the exercise less dynamic.

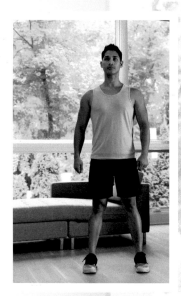

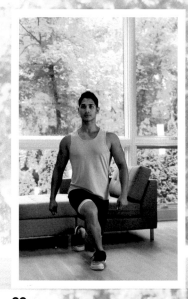

01 Stand tall with your hands by your sides and feet shoulder-width apart.

02 Cross your left leg behind your right and lunge as far as you can to the right. Landing on your heel, bend both legs and sit as low into the lunge as possible.

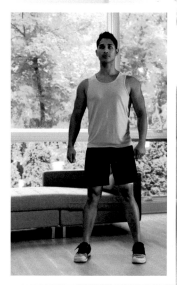

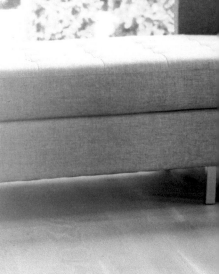

03 Press through the heel of the front foot and straighten the body back to standing position, standing tall to engage the core.

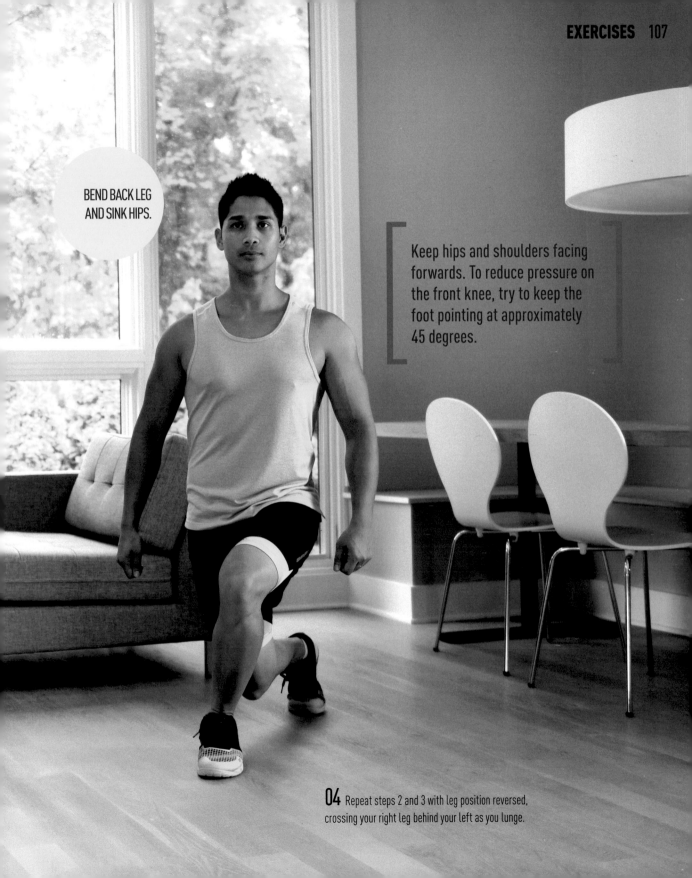

BEND BACK LEG
AND SINK HIPS.

Keep hips and shoulders facing
forwards. To reduce pressure on
the front knee, try to keep the
foot pointing at approximately
45 degrees.

04 Repeat steps 2 and 3 with leg position reversed,
crossing your right leg behind your left as you lunge.

ARCHER PULL-UP

These are the bridge between regular pull-ups and single-arm ones. The motion replicates drawing a bow to shoot an arrow, generating single-arm strength and power.

MORE DIFFICULT

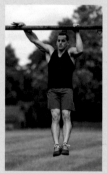

Modify speed: In step 3, slowly lower back down to the hanging position over a count of four to accentuate the eccentric muscle contraction and build power.

LESS DIFFICULT

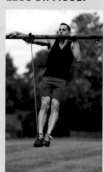

Modify stability: Use a resistance band, or place one foot on a chair, to increase stability and decrease the amount of weight being moved, and to provide assistance.

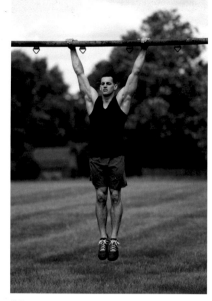

Avoid momentum, don't swing, and pay particular attention to the deceleration – the slow lowering or eccentric contraction – by controlling your descent.

01 Position yourself directly under the pull-up bar. Hop up and grab the bar with an overhand grip (palms facing away) wider than your shoulders. Hang from the bar with arms straight.

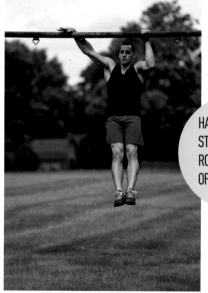

HAND OF STRAIGHT ARM ROLLS TO TOP OF BAR.

02 Pull yourself up to the left, tucking your left elbow tight to the chest so your right arm is extended across the width of the bar, parallel to the ground, at the top of the pull-up.

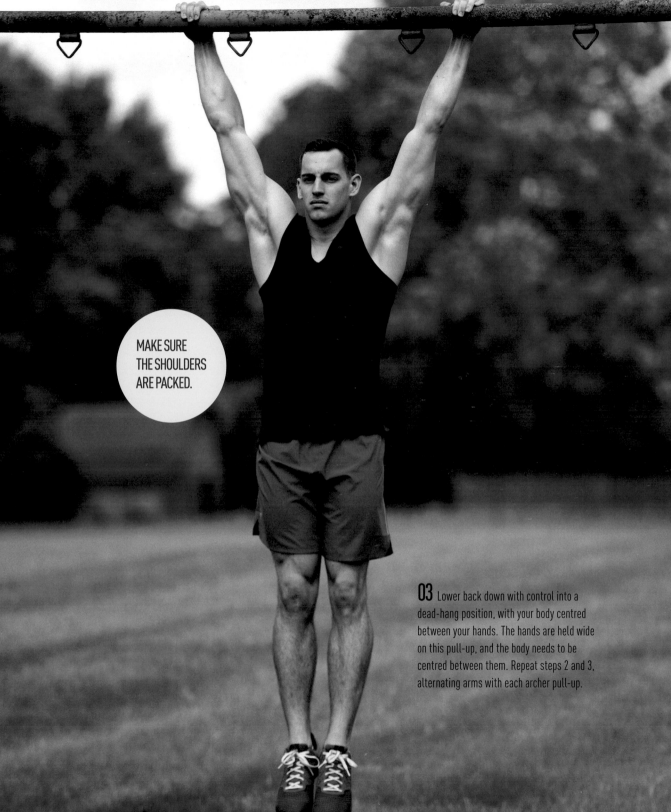

MAKE SURE
THE SHOULDERS
ARE PACKED.

03 Lower back down with control into a
dead-hang position, with your body centred
between your hands. The hands are held wide
on this pull-up, and the body needs to be
centred between them. Repeat steps 2 and 3,
alternating arms with each archer pull-up.

HANGING LEG RAISE

This is the Holy Grail of abdominal exercises. It will build a bulletproof core, increase grip strength and flexibility, and decompress your spine.

MORE DIFFICULT

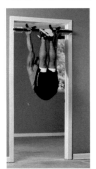

Modify range of motion: In step 2, bring your toes to touch the bar between your hands. This almost doubles the working range of the exercise and increases the work for abs, back, and hips.

LESS DIFFICULT

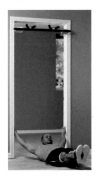

Modify points of contact: In preparation for eventually performing a hanging exercise, start practising leg raises on the floor to increase stability and focus on controlling the raising and lowering of the legs.

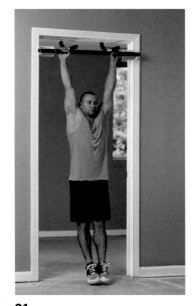

01 Stand directly under the pull-up bar. Hop up and grab the bar with an overhand grip (palms facing away), hands wider than shoulders, and hang with arms straight.

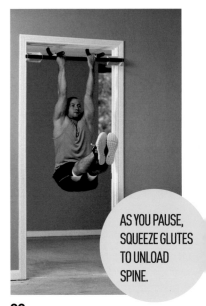

AS YOU PAUSE, SQUEEZE GLUTES TO UNLOAD SPINE.

02 With shoulders open and packed and legs kept straight, raise your legs with control until they're just beyond parallel to the floor. Pause for two seconds.

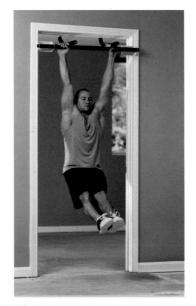

03 Lower your legs under control, and repeat.

FROG HOLD

Frog holds strengthen upper arms, forearms, and wrists. They also strengthen the abdominal muscles and improve balance and coordination for exercises such as planche holds.

MORE DIFFICULT

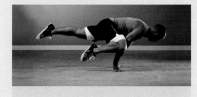

Modify points of contact: In step 2, extend one leg. This requires elevating more weight and challenges the core more intensely.

LESS DIFFICULT

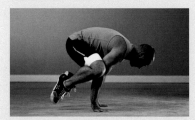

Modify points of contact: In step 2, move the knees to the outside of your arms to widen your base of support, making balancing easier.

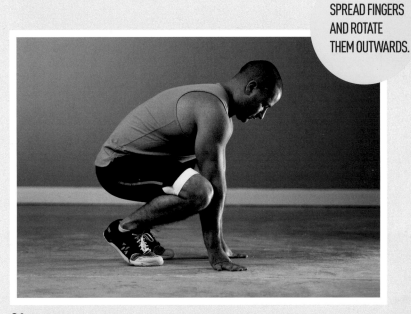

SPREAD FINGERS AND ROTATE THEM OUTWARDS.

01 Beginning in a crouched position, press your knees to the back of your arms, and lift onto the balls of your feet.

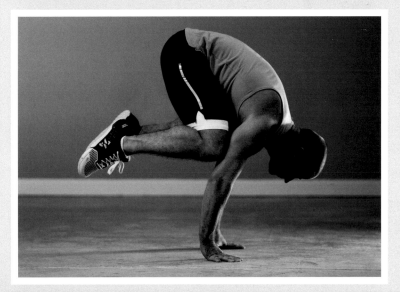

02 Transfer your weight to your upper body, lift your feet off of the floor, and hold.

FOREARM PRESS-UP

This exercise combines a forearm plank and press-up to work the chest, triceps, back, and core. This press-up is an excellent way to build strength for exercises such as the planche in Level 3.

MORE DIFFICULT

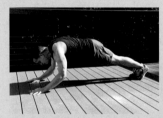

Modify speed: In step 3, lower the body slowly over a count of four to provide an eccentric muscle contraction that helps build strength and power.

LESS DIFFICULT

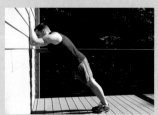

Modify body angle: Perform with hands against a wall to shift more weight into the stronger muscles of the lower body.

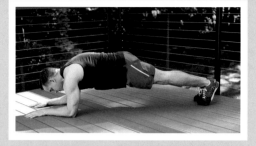

01 Start with forearms on the floor and legs extended, with the body evenly balanced between forearms and toes in a forearm plank position.

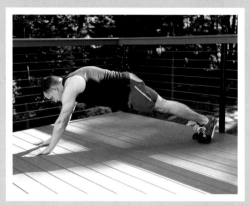

02 Push down evenly through the palms of your hands, raising your body as you fully straighten your arms.

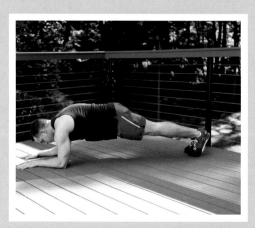

03 Slowly lower back down by bending the arms to return to the forearm plank starting position.

HANDS OPEN WITH PALMS FLAT ON FLOOR.

HOLLOW BODY HOLD

This killer abdominal exercise is essential to master because it teaches the posterior pelvic tilt required for exercises such as handstands.

MORE DIFFICULT

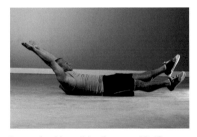

In step 2, add small leg flutters of 5–10cm (2–4in) to create greater engagement of your core.

LESS DIFFICULT

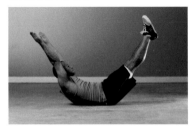

Modify body angle and range of motion: In step 2, hold legs higher to decrease leverage and the weight of the legs.

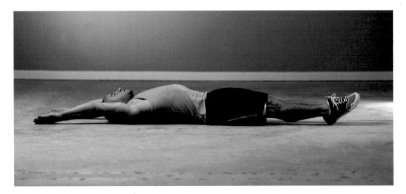

01 Lie on your back with arms and legs extended. Pull your belly button in and tuck your pelvis to connect your lower back to the floor.

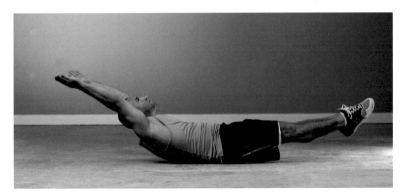

02 Slowly raise your legs, shoulders, and head off of the ground. Hold this curved position for the duration of the exercise.

KEEP LOWER BACK AGAINST FLOOR, ENGAGE ABS AND GLUTES.

T-STAND

Lengthen the hamstrings, learn to control the hips, and challenge your balance in this yoga-inspired functional exercise.

MORE DIFFICULT

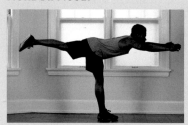

Modify stability and range of motion: In all steps, extend your arms overhead to lengthen your torso and challenge balance.

LESS DIFFICULT

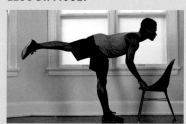

Modify stability: Hold a box, chair, or bench for balance so you can focus on keeping your hips square to the floor throughout the motion.

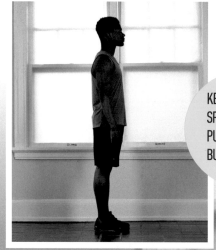

KEEP SPINE LONG, PULL BELLY BUTTON IN.

01 Stand with feet together and arms at your sides.

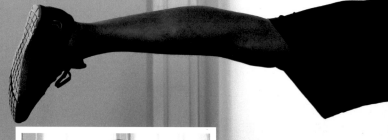

02 Inhale and slowly bend from the hips, lowering the torso and letting your arms hang. As you fold forwards, raise one leg until torso, arms, and leg are parallel to the floor.

03 Exhale as you lift the torso and lower the leg in one fluid motion. Repeat steps 2 and 3 with the opposite leg.

[
If balancing is a challenge, bend deeper at the waist to allow fingertips to touch the floor.
]

Try this ...

Adding a dynamic kick increases the range of motion and generates a force your core has to work to stabilize.

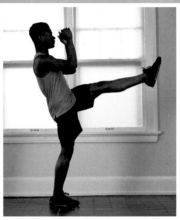

T-STAND KICK
As you stand tall in step 3, bring the back leg through and snap out a kick.

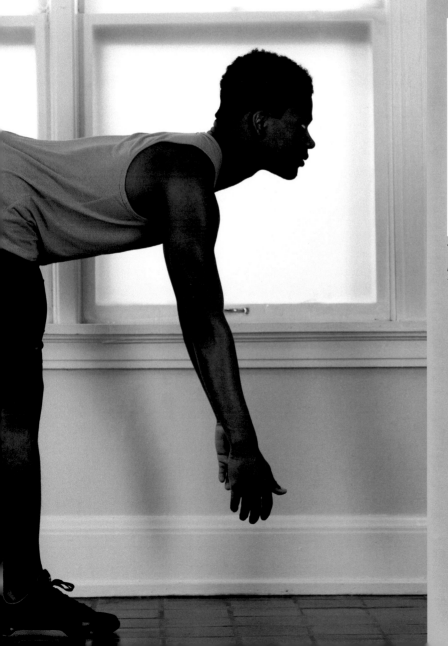

HANGING REVERSE CURL

This targets your lower abdominals and lower back. A strong, flexible core makes you more powerful in all endeavours.

MORE DIFFICULT

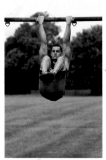

Modify range of motion and repetitions: In step 2, add a smaller second knee tuck/crunch at the top of the motion before fully straightening legs in step 3 increasing the work by 50 per cent.

LESS DIFFICULT

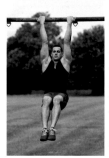

Modify range of motion: In step 2, tuck and raise the knees only until thighs are parallel to the ground to decrease the work for the knees and the time the core needs to be engaged.

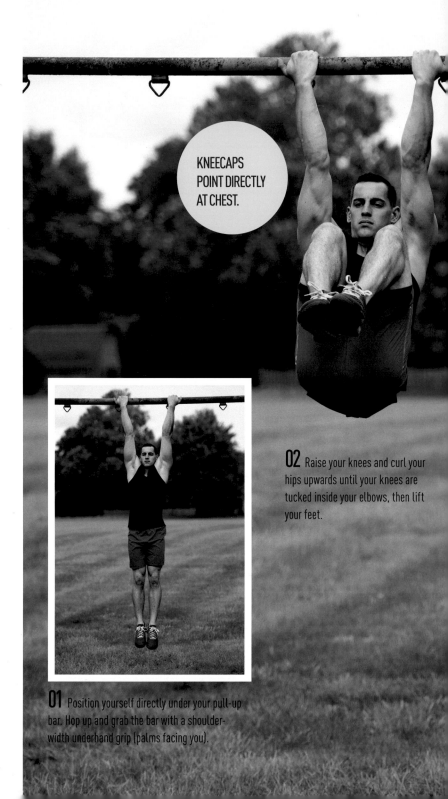

KNEECAPS POINT DIRECTLY AT CHEST.

02 Raise your knees and curl your hips upwards until your knees are tucked inside your elbows, then lift your feet.

01 Position yourself directly under your pull-up bar. Hop up and grab the bar with a shoulder-width underhand grip (palms facing you).

This exercise can be performed from a dead hang – hanging from the bar with arms straight and shoulders packed – but make sure you're not swinging and using momentum.

Try this ...

Twist both knees across the body as you curl upwards, as if skiing moguls, to engage the obliques.

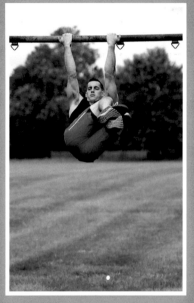

SKI TUCKS
Bring both knees across the body to one elbow, lower, and repeat to the opposite elbow.

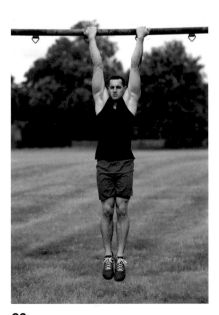

03 Lower back down slowly until your feet nearly touch the ground.

SHRIMP SQUAT

This unilateral leg exercise burns fat and increases strength, but it requires balance, core strength, and coordination – making it both fun and challenging.

MORE DIFFICULT

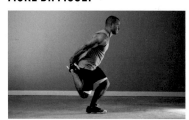

Modify stability: In steps 2, 3, and 4, hold the back leg with both hands to decrease balance and leverage, increasing the workload for the core, glutes, and legs.

LESS DIFFICULT

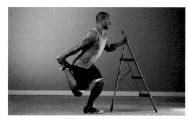

Modify stability: Hold any available prop for support, to slowly build strength with correct form.

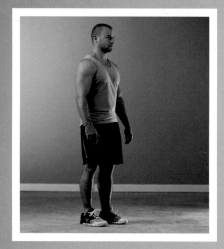

01 Stand with feet shoulder-width apart and hands at your sides.

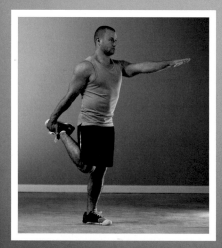

02 Bend one leg at the knee and reach back to hold the ankle with the same arm. Extend the other arm out straight for balance.

Try to maintain a rigid body throughout to retain energy. When a joint is unstable, the energy produced by your musculature can't be efficiently transferred through the body to produce optimal movements.

DON'T LET SQUATTING KNEE BUCKLE INWARDS.

03 Bend the front leg at the ankle, knee, then hip and, keeping the torso tall, lower your body into a squat until the knee of the backwards-bent leg hovers above or taps the floor.

04 Press through the heel of the front foot and straighten the body back to standing position, one ankle held and the other arm out straight for balance. Repeat steps 2 and 3, using the other side of the body.

BACK BRIDGE

Stretch the front of your body, strengthen the muscles supporting your spine, and work almost every muscle on the back of the body in this familiar and fun exercise.

MORE DIFFICULT

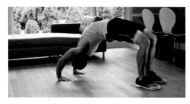

Modify range of motion: After reaching full extension in step 2, lower halfway, press back to full extension, and then lower completely.

LESS DIFFICULT

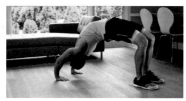

Modify speed: Instead of doing repetitions, hold the highest point of the exercise in step 2 for the duration.

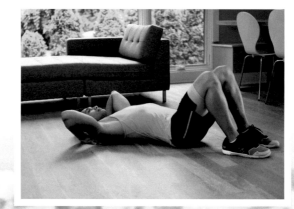

01 Lie on your back on the floor with knees and elbows bent, palms on the floor by the side of your head, and fingers pointing at your toes.

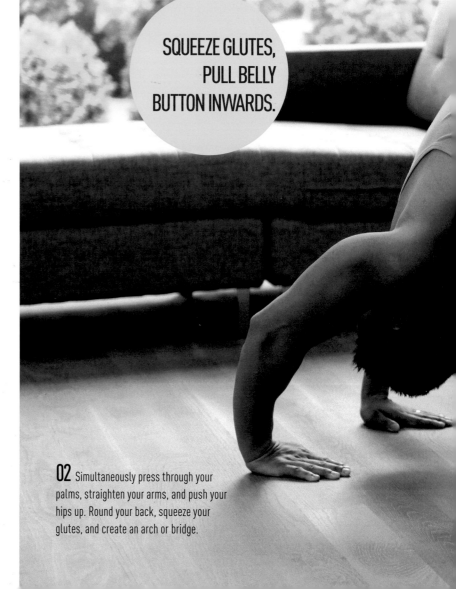

SQUEEZE GLUTES, PULL BELLY BUTTON INWARDS.

02 Simultaneously press through your palms, straighten your arms, and push your hips up. Round your back, squeeze your glutes, and create an arch or bridge.

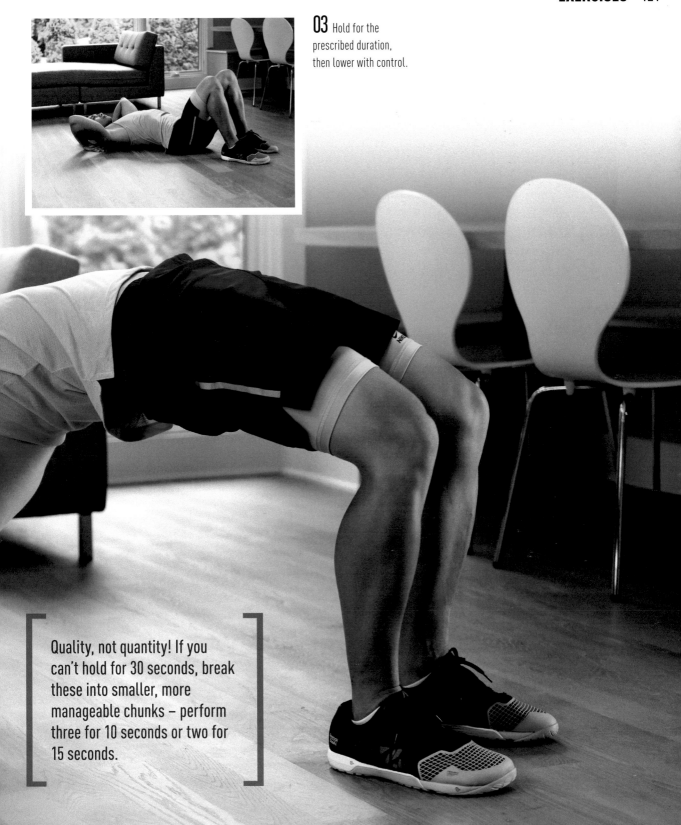

03 Hold for the prescribed duration, then lower with control.

Quality, not quantity! If you can't hold for 30 seconds, break these into smaller, more manageable chunks – perform three for 10 seconds or two for 15 seconds.

PIGEON PEEL

The peel in Level 1 increases strength in hips, hamstrings, glutes, and core. This version takes it further by rotating the legs, providing greater work for the gluteus medius and tensor fascia latae.

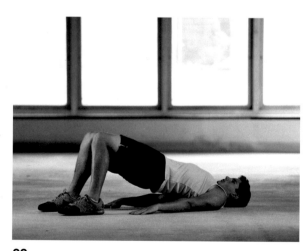

THE CLOSER THE HEELS TO THE GLUTES, THE HARDER.

01 Lie flat on your back on the floor or a mat. Bend your legs and place your feet on the floor wider than your shoulders. Roll your inner thighs together and squeeze them tight.

MORE DIFFICULT

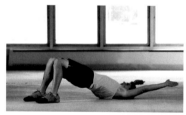

Modify points of contact: In step 2, extend and elevate the arms to remove any leverage, increasing the load on the glutes and core.

LESS DIFFICULT

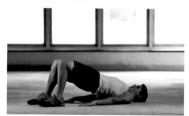

Modify speed: In step 2, hold at the top of the motion instead of performing repetitions, to create an isolation hold and build strength.

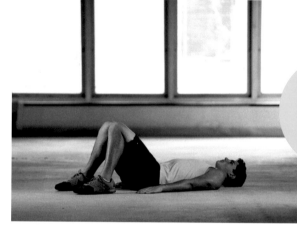

02 Press through the soles, squeeze the glutes, and lift the hips to form a straight line from shoulders to knees. Pause at the top and hold for one or two seconds before lowering back to the floor under control.

BUTTERFLY PEEL

The butterfly peel rotates the legs, providing greater work for the iliopsoas, sartorius, pectineus, and piriformis.

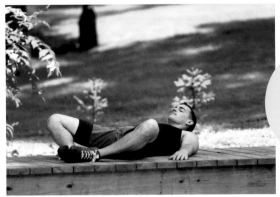

IT'S HARDER THE CLOSER THE HEELS ARE TO THE GLUTES.

01 Lie flat on your back on the ground. Bend your legs, place your feet on the ground with soles together, and open the knees as wide as possible.

MORE DIFFICULT

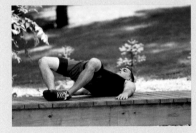

Modify stability: In step 2, after reaching the top of the motion, lower halfway, raise fully, then lower with control, for 1.5 reps.

LESS DIFFICULT

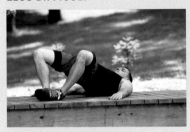

Modify speed: Hold at the top of the motion in step 2 instead of doing reps to create an isolation hold and build strength.

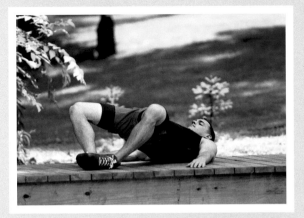

02 Press through the feet, squeeze the glutes, and lift the hips until your body forms a straight line from shoulders to open knees. Pause at the top of the motion and hold for one or two seconds before lowering back to the ground under control.

BULGARIAN SPLIT SQUAT

This unilateral leg exercise is incredibly useful as it not only builds leg strength, it also increases flexibility of hip flexors and helps to create overall balance.

MORE DIFFICULT

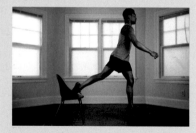

Modify range of motion: In step 2, add a plyometric jump to increase the workload and create performance-enhancing power.

LESS DIFFICULT

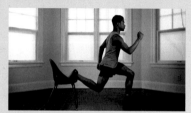

Modify speed: Hold in the deepest position of step 2 for the duration. This isolation hold will generate strength.

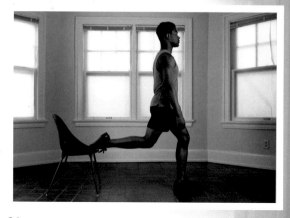

01 Stand with the top of your back foot on a bench, chair, or other elevated surface.

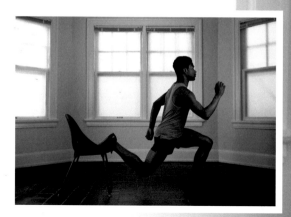

02 Bend your legs and lower body until the thigh of the front leg is parallel to the floor, and pause for two to three seconds.

Extend your arms out in front for balance, or overhead to increase the challenge.

THE HIGHER
THE BACK FOOT,
THE HARDER THE
EXERCISE.

03 Return to a standing position by pressing
through the heel of the front foot, standing tall
to engage the core.

1–2 PUSH

The 1–2 push is an intense, full-body move that will elevate your heart rate while working the muscles in your core, arms, and legs. Complete the move as quickly as you can, but that correct form takes priority.

MORE DIFFICULT

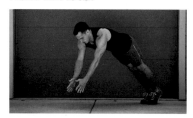

Modify range of motion: In step 3, add a plyometric (clap) press-up to generate explosive upper body power.

LESS DIFFICULT

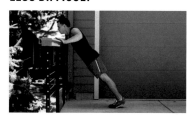

Modify body angle: For all steps, place your hands on a tall prop, shifting most of the weight into the lower body.

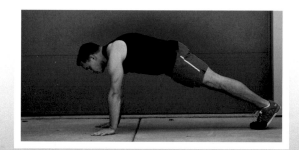

01 Begin in the plank position with hands on the floor slightly wider than shoulders, legs extended, and on your toes. Engage the core and form a straight line from ankles to head.

BRING KNEES COMPLETELY THROUGH ELBOWS.

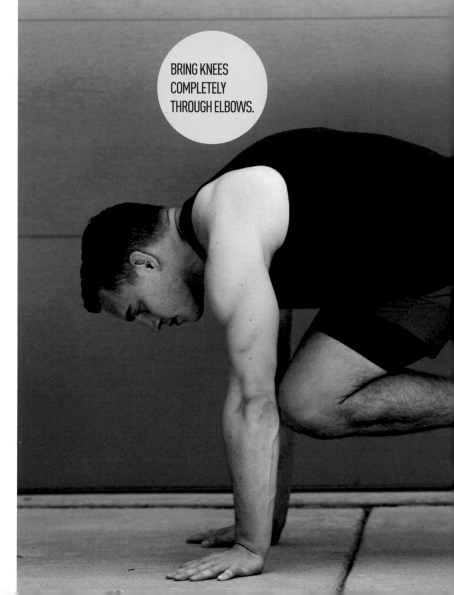

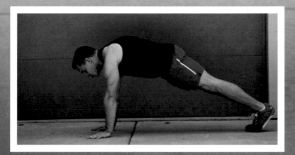

02 Bend your elbows, bringing the chest towards the floor until your elbows are bent slightly beyond 90 degrees.

03 Push up off of the floor and straighten the arms.

04 As arms reach full extension, bring your right knee to your chest and quickly switch legs, bringing the left knee to the chest. Then return to the starting position. Repeat steps 2 through 4, alternating legs.

Try this ...

By changing the angle of the legs when you bring the knee to the chest, you can create greater activation of the obliques.

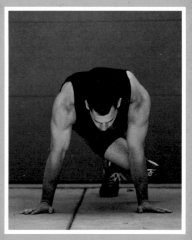

DIAGONAL MOUNTAIN CLIMBER
In the last step, take the knee across the body to the opposite elbow.

[Remember: form comes first, speed second.]

DRAGON WALK

This is not named after a character from *Game of Thrones* – but if you were going to crown one total-body exercise, this might be it. Dragon walks target so many muscle groups, that they may leave you breathing fire.

MORE DIFFICULT

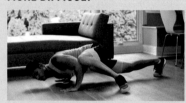

Modify speed: Add a pause at the bottom of each rep, forcing you to hold your weight in the most challenging position.

LESS DIFFICULT

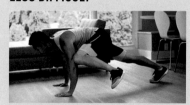

Modify range of motion: Keep your hands still and focus on only bringing the knees to the shoulders.

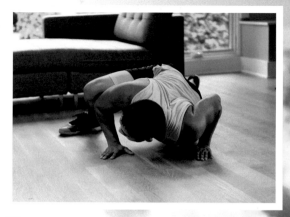

01 Assume a modified military press-up position, with your hands staggered, arms slightly bent, and right elbow touching the right knee.

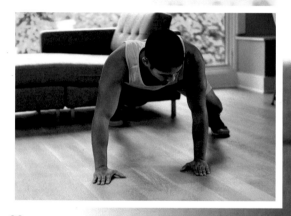

02 Straighten your arms and step forwards with your right hand and left foot as if crawling.

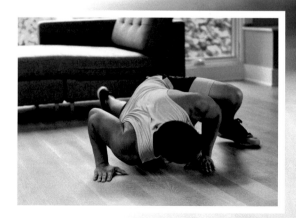

03 Drop back into the modified or staggered military press-up position, this time with the left elbow touching the left knee.

Think like a reptile: Stay low to the ground as you move with smooth, gliding, controlled steps. Slink across the floor.

CHIN UP, EYES FORWARDS.

04 Repeat steps 2 and 3, continuing to crawl forwards in incremental controlled steps for the duration.

SKATER JUMP

This exercise mimics the movement of a speed skater zooming across the ice. Skater jumps will strengthen your legs while improving balance and coordination.

MORE DIFFICULT

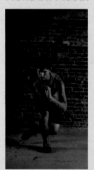

Modify range of motion: In step 3, land and perform a one-legged squat, hold the position for a count of three, and switch sides. This takes away momentum, forcing you to engage quads, glutes, and core.

LESS DIFFICULT

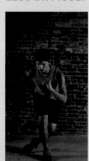

Modify points of contact: As you land in step 3, allow the back leg to touch the floor for balance and stability, allowing you to focus on the depth of the exercise without fear of falling.

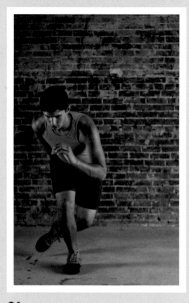

01 Stand with your right knee slightly bent and all your weight on that foot. Cross your left foot behind your right ankle and lower into a half squat.

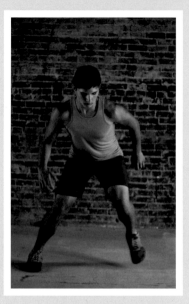

02 Bound to the left by pushing off your right foot. As you do, swing your arms across your body in the direction of your jump.

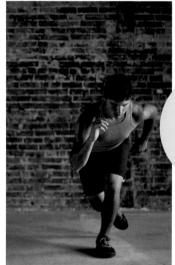

MOVE FROM SIDE TO SIDE IN A FLUID MOTION.

03 Land on your left foot and bring the right foot behind your left. Repeat steps 2 and 3, reversing feet so you begin by standing on your left foot.

ARCHER PRESS-UP

You'll place the majority of the weight on one side, forcing you to hold more of your weight with one arm. This generates strength and stability for chest, shoulder, back, and triceps.

MORE DIFFICULT

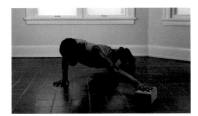

Modify range of motion: Elevate your extended arm on a prop, increasing the activation of the chest, shoulder, and arm.

LESS DIFFICULT

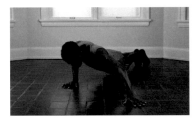

Modify points of contact: Move the extended arm closer to the body to create greater leverage to assist the press-up.

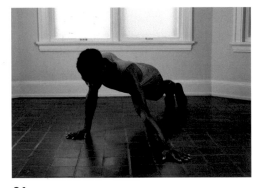

01 Begin in a modified military press-up, core engaged, balanced between toes and hands, in a straight line from ankles to head, with your left arm out straight from the body.

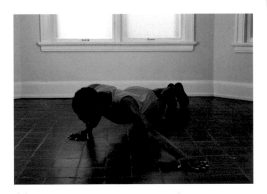

02 Bend the right elbow, keeping it tight against the ribcage, and lower your chest with control towards the floor. Pause at the bottom.

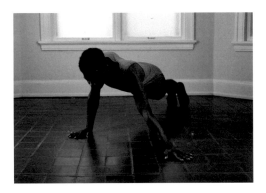

03 Push up through the right arm to return to the starting position. Repeat the exercise with opposite arm.

THE STABILIZING ARM WORKS AS LITTLE AS POSSIBLE.

BACKWARDS PRESS-UP

The core-killing backwards press-up is not for the faint of heart. Adding a fast, explosive drive or push with the legs makes your core contract to slow and stabilize the body.

MORE DIFFICULT

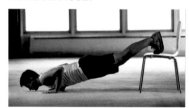

Modify body angle: Place feet on a chair or other prop to shift more weight into the upper body and cause the shoulders, chest, and core to work harder.

LESS DIFFICULT

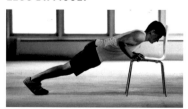

Modify body angle: Elevate hands on a prop and perform inclined military press-ups to increase stability while building core and shoulder strength.

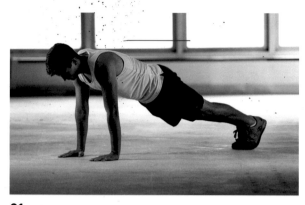

01 Begin in a plank position.

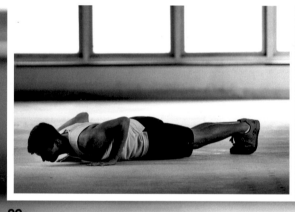

02 Bend your elbows, lowering into a military press-up. Keep your core tight and body flat.

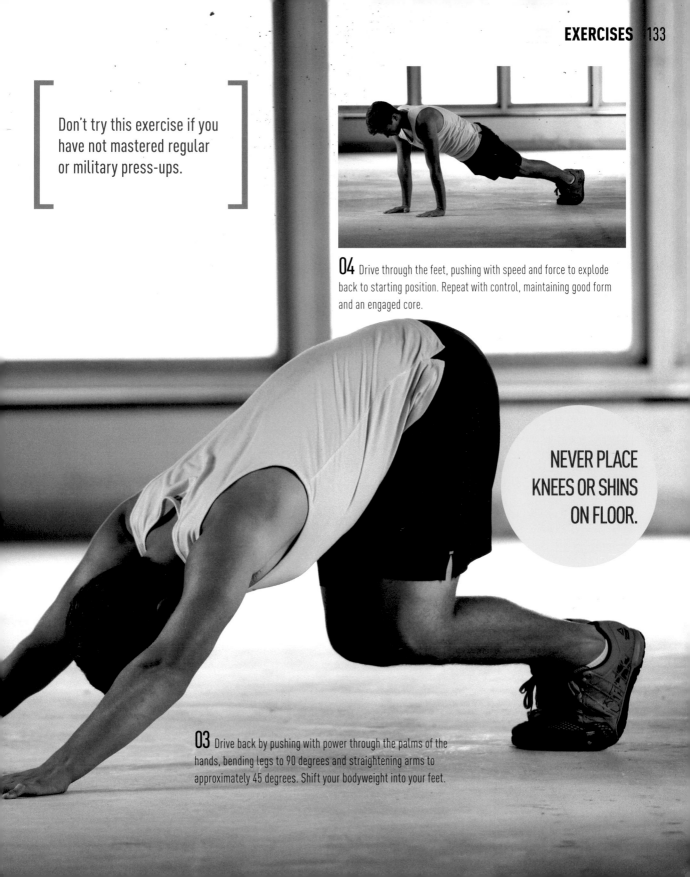

Don't try this exercise if you have not mastered regular or military press-ups.

04 Drive through the feet, pushing with speed and force to explode back to starting position. Repeat with control, maintaining good form and an engaged core.

NEVER PLACE KNEES OR SHINS ON FLOOR.

03 Drive back by pushing with power through the palms of the hands, bending legs to 90 degrees and straightening arms to approximately 45 degrees. Shift your bodyweight into your feet.

SINGLE-LEG BURPEE

Raising a leg throughout the plank and press-up phase of the Burpee adds an increased load for the core, challenging the abdominals, lower back, and stabilizing leg.

MORE DIFFICULT

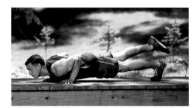

Modify points of contact: In steps 1 through 4, change the hands for the press-up to a military press-up position.

LESS DIFFICULT

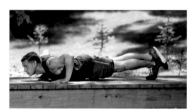

Modify points of contact: In steps 2 and 3, cross the elevated leg on top of the stabilizing one, adding support and increasing balance.

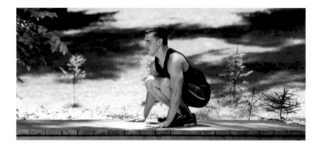

01 With your feet hip-width apart, bend your knees and bring your hands to the ground just in front of your feet.

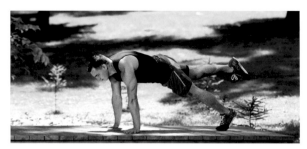

02 Hop your feet back into a plank position with one leg elevated to hip height.

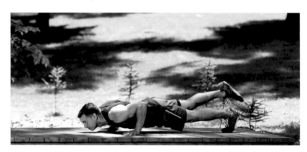

03 Perform one press-up with your core engaged and leg elevated.

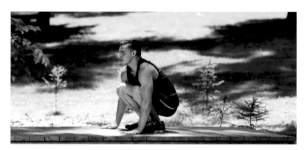

04 Lower the raised leg and jump your feet back to your hands, shifting your weight into the heels and lifting your chest.

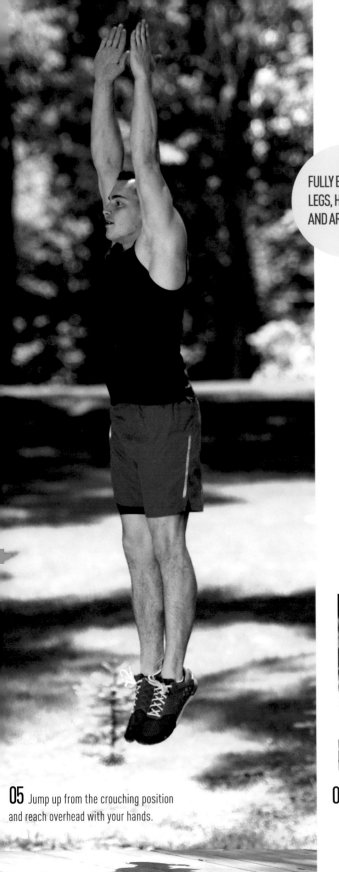

FULLY EXTEND LEGS, HIPS, AND ARMS.

The Burpee was created in the 1930s by American physiologist Royal Huddleston Burpee for a PhD thesis. Burpees are a total-body strength and cardiovascular exercise.

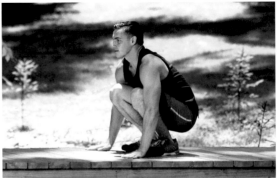

05 Jump up from the crouching position and reach overhead with your hands.

06 Land softly with a slight bend at your knees, hips, and ankles.

PLYOMETRIC PRESS-UP

Adding an explosive plyometric press and controlled landing to the press-up – the perfect compound exercise – will generate incredible upper-body power.

MORE DIFFICULT

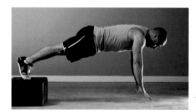

Modify body angle: For all steps, place feet on a stable elevated surface, shifting weight to the upper body so it works harder.

LESS DIFFICULT

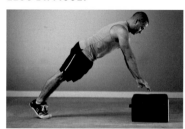

Modify body angle: Place your hands on a stable elevated prop, shifting weight to the lower body so the upper body has less work to perform.

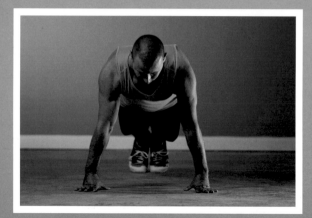

01 Begin in a full plank or regular press-up position with core engaged, balancing between toes and hands, and forming a straight line from ankles to head.

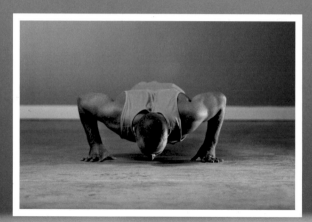

02 With core still engaged, bend your elbows, bringing your chest towards the floor.

Landing with arms straight would be harmful. Instead, land immediately into the next rep, bending elbows and wrists.

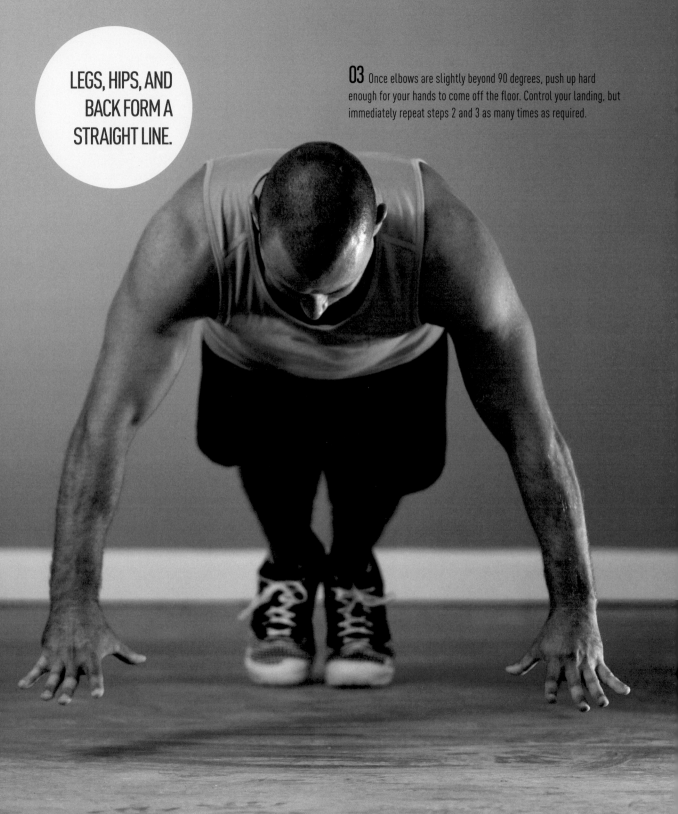

LEGS, HIPS, AND
BACK FORM A
STRAIGHT LINE.

03 Once elbows are slightly beyond 90 degrees, push up hard
enough for your hands to come off the floor. Control your landing, but
immediately repeat steps 2 and 3 as many times as required.

STOP-AND-GO PRESS-UP

Pausing at the bottom portion of the press-up forces you to recruit as many motor units (muscle fibres) as possible to overcome the weight. Pausing at any other point builds isometric strength.

MORE DIFFICULT

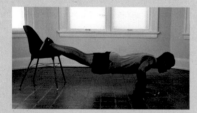

Modify body angle: Use a chair or prop to elevate your feet and transfer weight into the upper body and core to work them harder.

LESS DIFFICULT

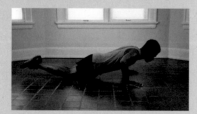

Modify body angle: Kneel to transfer your weight to the lower body, decreasing the work required from the upper body.

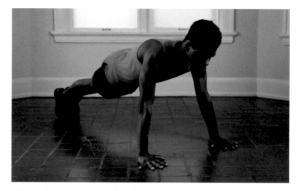

01 Assume a full plank or traditional press-up position with the body balanced between toes and hands, and with the hands slightly wider than the shoulders.

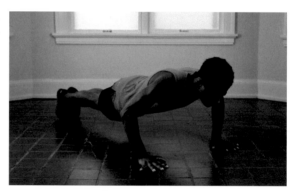

02 Bend your legs and lower the body until the thigh of the front leg is parallel to the floor, and pause for two to three seconds.

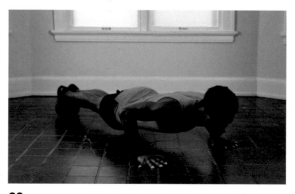

03 Continue to lower to the deepest part of the press-up and hold for two seconds.

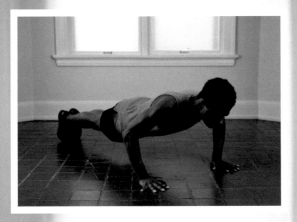

04 Press through the palms to straighten the arms and lift the chest. At the halfway point, pause and hold for two seconds.

Stop-and-go press-ups activate more muscle fibres than their standard counterparts, allowing greater gains in strength in a shorter period of time.

05 Return to the starting position with arms fully straightened.

USE THIS TECHNIQUE WITH ANY TYPE OF PRESS-UP.

PIKE PRESS-UP TO PRESS-UP

Build boulder shoulders with this press-up combo that also engages the core and lower body.

MORE DIFFICULT

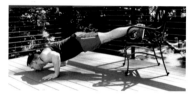

Modify body angle: Elevate feet to transfer mass to the upper body, requiring it to perform more work.

LESS DIFFICULT

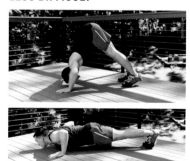

Modify stability: Perform the press-ups separately. This lets you focus on depth and form.

When you perform press-ups, imagine rotating the palms as if screwing them into the floor. This will lock your shoulders and create joint stability.

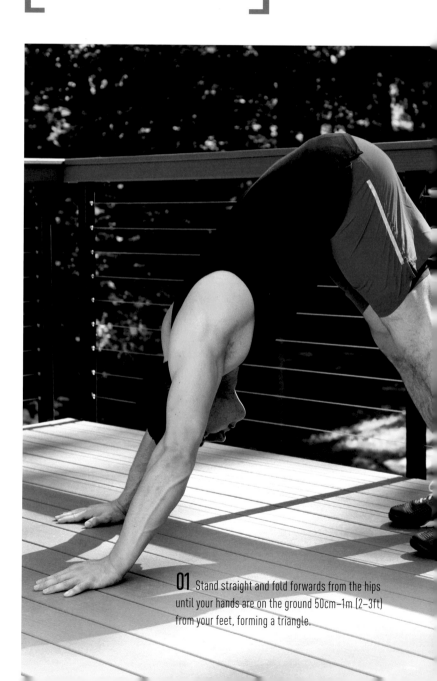

01 Stand straight and fold forwards from the hips until your hands are on the ground 50cm–1m (2–3ft) from your feet, forming a triangle.

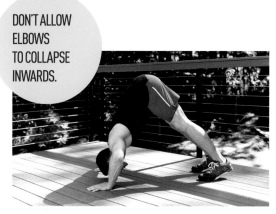

DON'T ALLOW ELBOWS TO COLLAPSE INWARDS.

02 Perform a pike press-up by bending your arms to lower the crown of the head to the ground. Your arms should form a 90-degree angle.

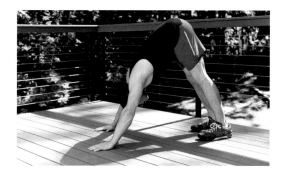

03 Straighten the arms and press away from the ground, returning to the pike position.

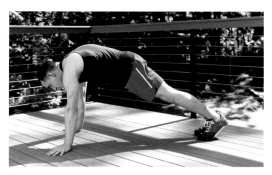

04 Walk the hands away from the feet until you form a plank or standard press-up position, with hands slightly wider than shoulders.

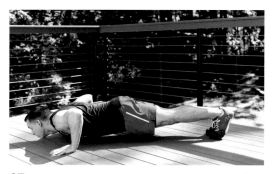

05 Perform a standard press-up by bending elbows to lower the body until your nose touches the ground.

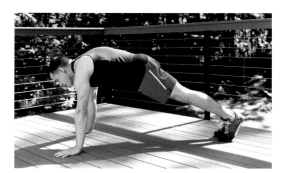

06 Straighten the arms, pressing through the centre of the palms to return to the plank or standard press-up position.

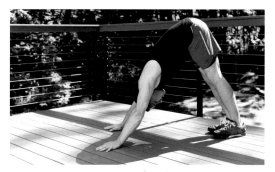

07 Walk the hands back towards the feet, returning to the pike position.

CRAZY 8s

There are any number of rep schemes you can follow when working out, but one of the absolute best I have ever used to gain strength and power is affectionately known as "Crazy 8s" in my gym. It consists of eight rounds of an exercise, performing just five reps followed by a 30-second to one-minute rest. This low-rep but high-volume style of training will build your strength and help you gain muscle.

Avoid working to failure in the latter sets or on very challenging exercises such as shrimp squats. If three or four reps is your max with good form, stop at that point and rest.

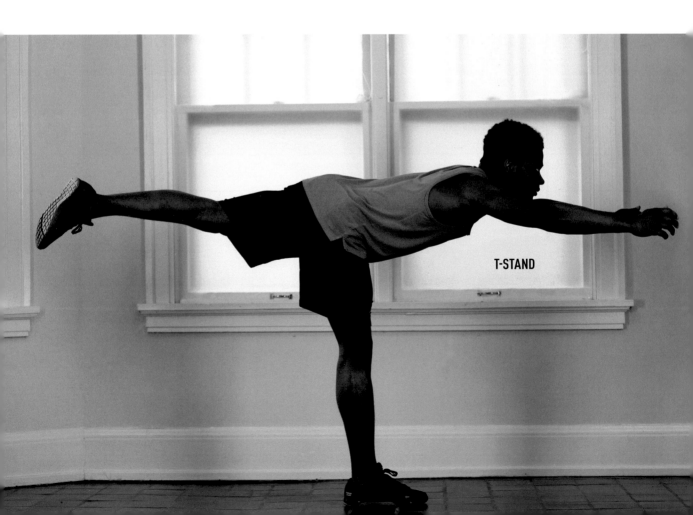

T-STAND

Perform 5 reps of each exercise followed by a rest of 30 seconds to one minute, depending on your strength and endurance. Perform eight rounds of the exercise (40 reps in total), before moving on to the next exercise.

DEEP SQUAT

work 5 reps, rest 0:30–1:00	**P**102

↻ REPEAT for eight rounds

SHRIMP SQUAT

work 5 reps, rest 0:30–1:00	**P**118

↻ REPEAT for a total of eight rounds – four rounds per leg, alternate each round

T-STAND

work 5 reps, rest 0:30–1:00	**P**114

↻ REPEAT for a total of eight rounds – four rounds per leg, alternate each round

ALTERNATING CROSS-OVER LUNGE

work 5 reps, rest 0:30–1:00	**P**106

↻ REPEAT for a total of eight rounds – four rounds per leg, alternate each round

PIGEON PEEL

work 5 reps, rest 0:30–1:00	**P**122

↻ REPEAT for eight rounds

BUTTERFLY PEEL

work 5 reps, rest 0:30–1:00	**P**123

↻ REPEAT for eight rounds

BULGARIAN SPLIT SQUAT

work 5 reps, rest 0:30–1:00	**P**124

↻ REPEAT for a total of eight rounds – four rounds per leg, alternate each round

CORE POWER

Perform all exercises in order, then rest 30 seconds. Complete four rounds.

HANGING LEG RAISE

10x	**P**110

HOLLOW BODY HOLD

0:30	**P**113

HANGING REVERSE CURL

10x	**P**116

BACK BRIDGE

0:30	**P**120

🕐 REST 0:30

↻ REPEAT Core Power for a total of four rounds

HERCULES WORKOUT

Roman hero Hercules is famous for his strength. This workout features a pyramid format of decreasing reps and introduces multiplanar motions and unilateral exercises to challenge the foundation you built in Level 1.

Perform each set for five rounds, subtracting one rep per round where shown (pyramid format). Rest 30 seconds between rounds. Perform all sets and their exercises in order.

 SET A

BULGARIAN SPLIT SQUAT

10x each leg	P124

SPIDERMAN PRESS-UP

5x, 4x, 3x, 2x, 1x	P103

ARCHER PULL-UP

5x, 4x, 3x, 2x, 1x	P108

🕐 REST 0:30 after each round of the set
🔁 REPEAT for five rounds in pyramid format

 SET B

ALTERNATING CROSS-OVER LUNGE

10x each leg	P106

FOREARM PRESS-UP

5x, 4x, 3x, 2x, 1x	P112

CHIN-UP

5x, 4x, 3x, 2x, 1x	P050

🕐 REST 0:30 after each round of the set
🔁 REPEAT for five rounds in pyramid format

 SET C

PIGEON PEEL

10x	P122

BUTTERFLY PEEL

10x	P123

PIKE PRESS-UP TO PRESS-UP

5x, 4x, 3x, 2x, 1x	P140

INVERTED BODYWEIGHT ROW

5x, 4x, 3x, 2x, 1x	P054

🕐 REST 0:30 after each round of the set
🔁 REPEAT for five rounds in pyramid format
🔁 **REPEAT sets A–C for a total of three rounds**

FINISHER

Perform all exercises in order and repeat for three rounds with no rest between rounds.

1–2 PUSH

10x	P126

SKATER JUMP

20x	P130

SINGLE-LEG BURPEE

30x	P134

MOUNTAIN CLIMBER

40x	P042

🔁 REPEAT finisher for a total of three rounds

This is an AsFAP (As Fast As Possible) finisher, but remember to focus on form first, speed second. Push as hard as you can to boost your metabolism and improve your calorie burn.

HANNIBAL
WORKOUT

Hannibal is regarded as one of the greatest military leaders in history. He's best known for marching an army – including elephants – across the Alps. The same dogged determination and "nothing is impossible" attitude will be required to survive three rounds of this total body workout.

[Adding a stop-and-go or plyometrics changes the speed and force of an exercise, making it harder but also requiring the use of different types of muscle fibres.]

FINISHER

Perform all three exercises in order, then rest 30 seconds. Repeat for a total of five rounds. Total exercise time: 10 minutes.

Perform three full rounds with no rest between exercises or rounds.

DEEP SQUAT	
15x	**P**102

STOP-AND-GO PRESS-UP	
submax*	**P**138

T-STAND	
12x each leg	**P**114

ARCHER PULL-UP	
submax*	**P**108

PLYOMETRIC PRESS-UP	
submax*	**P**136

HANGING LEG RAISE	
10x	**P**110

↻ REPEAT the set for a total of three rounds

*Submax = 80 per cent of your max number of reps. If you're unsure of your max number of reps, perform the first round to failure (max) and subsequent rounds to 80 per cent of that max number – e.g., max = 10 reps, submax = 8 reps.

SINGLE-LEG BURPEE – LEFT	
work 0:20, rest 0:10	**P**134

SKATER JUMP	
work 0:20, rest 0:10	**P**130

SINGLE-LEG BURPEE – RIGHT	
work 0:20, rest 0:10	**P**134

🕐 REST 0:30
↻ REPEAT the finisher for a total of five rounds

PUSH-PULL PAIRS

This workout pairs exercises that complement each other by working opposing forces. Performing a push movement followed by a pull movement makes the workout more efficient because the change of direction helps avoid muscle strain and helps you to keep going for longer without the need for long rests.

If 10 reps are too many on any exercise, make things easier to allow you to continue. For example, for press-ups, drop to your knees and finish the remaining reps.

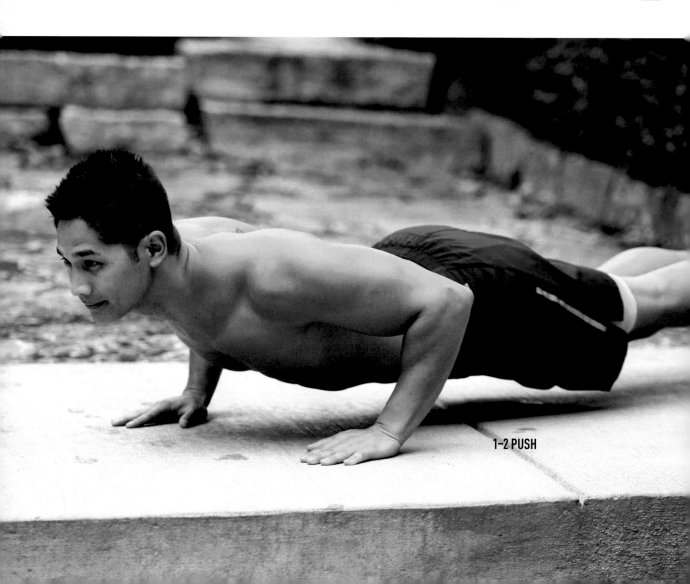

1–2 PUSH

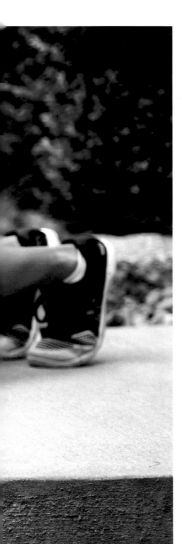

Perform each set for five rounds, subtracting two reps per round (pyramid format). Rest 30 seconds between rounds. Perform all sets and their exercises in order.

SET A

BACKWARDS PRESS-UP

10x, 8x, 6x, 4x, 2x	P132

ARCHER PULL-UP

10x, 8x, 6x, 4x, 2x	P108

🕒 REST 0:30 after each round of the set
↻ REPEAT for five rounds in pyramid format

SET B

STOP-AND-GO PRESS-UP

10x, 8x, 6x, 4x, 2x	P138

INVERTED BODYWEIGHT ROW

10x, 8x, 6x, 4x, 2x	P054

🕒 REST 0:30 after each round of the set
↻ REPEAT for five rounds in pyramid format

SET C

1–2 PUSH

10x, 8x, 6x, 4x, 2x	P126

CHIN-UP

10x, 8x, 6x, 4x, 2x	P050

🕒 REST 0:30 after each round of the set
↻ REPEAT for five rounds in pyramid format

HANGING REVERSE CURL

work 0:20, rest 0:10	P116

BURPEE

work 0:20, rest 0:10	P060

1–2 PUSH

work 0:20, rest 0:10	P126

HANGING LEG RAISE

work 0:20, rest 0:10	P110

↻ REPEAT Rip It for two rounds
🕒 REST 1:00
↻ REPEAT Rip It for two more rounds
🕒 REST 1:00

RIP IT

Perform all exercises in order for a total of four rounds, with a one-minute rest halfway through and at the end. Total exercise time: 10 minutes.

YUE FEI WORKOUT

Celebrated Chinese military mastermind Yue Fei personally fought in 126 battles and never lost a single engagement. An unbeatable mindset will be required to endure this gruelling total body workout. Multi-muscle compound exercises combined with multiplanar and unilateral exercises will keep your body off balance, increasing athletic performance while also forging strength and burning calories.

If you are struggling to perform the full number of reps for a Level 2 exercise, do as many reps as you can with good form and then switch to a Level 1 exercise to finish the reps. For example, swap the Level 2 archer pull-up for a Level 1 pull-up. This will help you to continue instead of simply stopping.

Perform three full rounds with no rest between exercises or rounds.

DEEP SQUAT	
15x	P102
SPIDERMAN PRESS-UP	
submax*	P103
BULGARIAN SPLIT SQUAT	
15x	P124
ARCHER PULL-UP	
submax*	P108
SINGLE-LEG BURPEE	
10x	P134
HOLLOW BODY HOLD	
0:30	P113

↻ REPEAT for a total of three rounds

*Submax = 80 per cent of your max number of reps. To calculate your max number of reps, perform the first round to failure (max) and subsequent rounds to 80 per cent of that max number – e.g., max = 10 reps, submax = 8 reps.

FINISHER
Perform four rounds for a total time of eight minutes.

HANGING LEG RAISE	
work 0:20, rest 0:10	P110
BURPEE	
work 0:20, rest 0:10	P060
HANGING REVERSE CURL	
work 0:20, rest 0:10	P116
MOUNTAIN CLIMBER	
work 0:20, rest 0:10	P043

↻ REPEAT for a total of four rounds

SUPER CIRCUIT FANTASTIC FOUR

Want the body of a comic book hero? This super circuit combines strength and speed by fusing a muscle-building bodyweight strength workout with a high-intensity interval-style set for maximum results.

To add variety or challenge to this workout, perform A + A (strength-oriented sets) followed by B + B (cardiovascular HIIT sets).

Perform two rounds of set 1 (A + B) with no rest between rounds, followed by two rounds of set 2 (A + B).

SET 1

A

SHRIMP SQUAT	
5x	**P**118

T-STAND	
10x	**P**114

STOP-AND-GO PRESS-UP	
10x	**P**138

ARCHER PULL-UP	
10x	**P**108

B

BACKWARDS PRESS-UP	
work 0:20, rest 0:10	**P**132

SKATER JUMP	
work 0:20, rest 0:10	**P**130

FRONT LUNGE	
work 0:20, rest 0:10	**P**104

DRAGON WALK	
work 0:20, rest 0:10	**P**128

↻ REPEAT set 1 for a total of two rounds

SET 2

A

FOREARM PRESS-UP	
10x	**P**112

HANGING REVERSE CURL	
10x	**P**116

DEEP SQUAT	
10x	**P**102

CHIN-UP	
10x	**P**050

B

1–2 PUSH	
work 0:20, rest 0:10	**P**126

HANGING LEG RAISE	
work 0:20, rest 0:10	**P**110

DRAGON WALK	
work 0:20, rest 0:10	**P**128

FROG HOLD	
work 0:20, rest 0:10	**P**110

↻ REPEAT set 2 for a total of two rounds

LEGENDARY LEGS

Multiple planes of motion, unilateral exercises, and the clock all combine to challenge you in this lower body workout. Focus on quality over quantity for incredible strength gains, which will also lead to increased power and athletic performance.

Perform the first round to max reps and then try to aim for 80 per cent of your max reps in the following three rounds. For example, if your max is 15 lunges in 30 seconds, aim for around 12 lunges while slowing the reps down to meet the 30-second time. This will ensure you can complete all four rounds.

Perform each set in order with no rest between exercises. Rest 30 seconds after each set. Complete four rounds for a total time of 20 minutes.

SET A

FRONT LUNGE	
0:30	P104

ALTERNATING CROSS-OVER LUNGE	
0:30	P106

SHRIMP SQUAT	
0:30	P118

DEEP SQUAT	
0:30	P102

🕐 REST 0:30 before set B

SET B

T-STAND	
0:30	P114

PIGEON PEEL	
0:30	P122

BUTTERFLY PEEL	
0:30	P123

BACK BRIDGE	
0:30	P120

🕐 REST 0:30

↻ REPEAT sets A–B for a total of four rounds

ALL-IN

Are you all-in? This workout is going to test your mental resolve as much as your physical prowess. Each exercise has a lower number of reps, allowing you to accomplish each with good form. The speed at which you perform the exercises and the rest after each is up to you. Can you go three rounds with no rest?

Don't perform half reps – all-in or modify! If you know you can't complete 10 archer pull-ups, perform as many complete reps as possible and then either assist with a chair or perform any easier pull such as standard pull-ups or inverted rows.

RIP IT
Perform all exercises in order for a total of four rounds, with a one-minute rest halfway through and at the end. Total exercise time: 10 minutes.

Try to rest as little as possible between exercises. Rest one minute after each round, and complete three rounds.

SHRIMP SQUAT	
5x per leg	P118

DEEP SQUAT	
20x	P102

FRONT LUNGE	
20x – 10 per leg	P104

SINGLE-LEG BURPEE	
20x – 10 per leg	P134

PIKE PRESS-UP TO PRESS-UP	
10x	P140

ARCHER PULL-UP	
10x	P108

DIP	
10x	P073

CHIN-UP	
10x	P050

HOLLOW BODY HOLD	
0:30 seconds	P113

🕐 REST 1:00
🔁 REPEAT the set for a total of three rounds

HANGING REVERSE CURL	
work 0:20, rest 0:10	P116

BURPEE	
work 0:20, rest 0:10	P060

1–2 PUSH	
work 0:20, rest 0:10	P126

HANGING LEG RAISE	
work 0:20, rest 0:10	P110

🔁 REPEAT Rip It for two rounds
🕐 REST 1:00
🔁 REPEAT Rip It for two more rounds
🕐 REST 1:00

FIRE

It's time to light a fire under you! This workout is a metabolic powerhouse, utilizing high-intensity intervals and multi-muscle compound exercises to torch body fat and build lean muscle. Your aim during each 20 seconds of work is to reach 80–90 per cent of your maximum heart rate.

At 80–90 per cent of maximum heart rate you should feel slightly uncomfortable, unable to hold a conversation, out of breath, and in need of each 10-second rest.

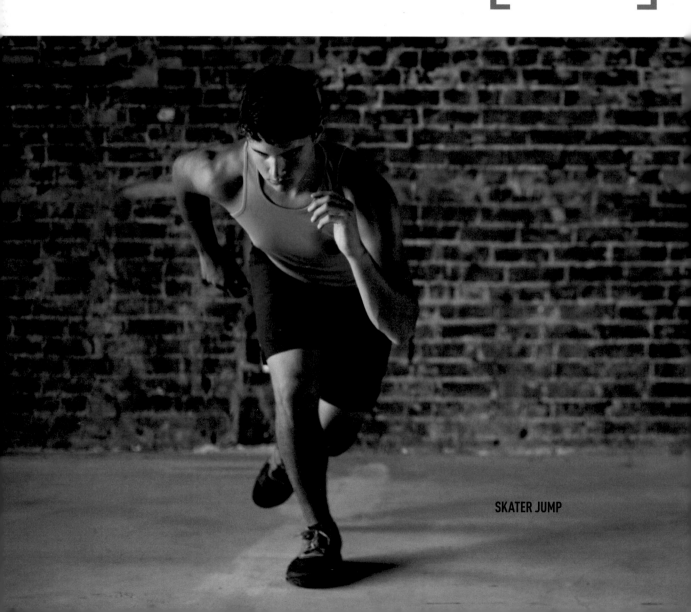

SKATER JUMP

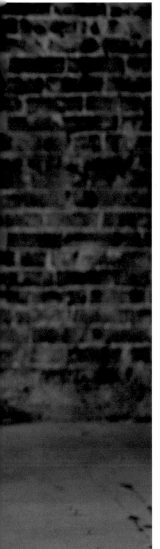

Perform each set for three rounds, followed by one minute rest, before moving on to the next set. Total exercise time: 21 minutes.

1–2 PUSH

| work 0:20, rest 0:10 | **P**126 |

SINGLE-LEG BURPEE – RIGHT

| work 0:20, rest 0:10 | **P**134 |

ARCHER PULL-UP

| work 0:20, rest 0:10 | **P**108 |

SINGLE-LEG BURPEE – LEFT

| work 0:20, rest 0:10 | **P**134 |

↻ REPEAT the set for a total of three rounds
🕐 REST 1:00 before set B

BACKWARDS PRESS-UP

| work 0:20, rest 0:10 | **P**132 |

SKATER JUMP

| work 0:20, rest 0:10 | **P**130 |

DEEP SQUAT

| work 0:20, rest 0:10 | **P**102 |

T-STAND

| work 0:20, rest 0:10 | **P**114 |

↻ REPEAT the set for a total of three rounds
🕐 REST 1:00 before set C

BULGARIAN SPLIT SQUAT – RIGHT

| work 0:20, rest 0:10 | **P**124 |

PLYOMETRIC PRESS-UP

| work 0:20, rest 0:10 | **P**136 |

BULGARIAN SPLIT SQUAT – LEFT

| work 0:20, rest 0:10 | **P**124 |

DRAGON WALK

| work 0:20, rest 0:10 | **P**128 |

↻ REPEAT the set for a total of three rounds
🕐 REST 1:00

TRI-PHASE

A phase is a distinct period or stage in a process of change, or a part of something's development. Each triplet in this workout features exercises geared to sculpt lean muscle, build strength, burn fat, and evolve your body.

Perform each set for three rounds, followed by one minute rest, before moving on to the next set.

 SET A

BULGARIAN SPLIT SQUAT	
15x each side	P124

STOP-AND GO PRESS-UP	
10x	P138

1–2 PUSH	
0:45	P126

↻ REPEAT the set for a total of three rounds
◷ REST 1:00 before set B

[For an added challenge, remove the rest between sets and perform all sets in order (A–D), repeating them three times.]

 SET B

T-STAND	
15x	P114

ARCHER PRESS-UP	
10x	P131

SKATER JUMP	
0:45	P130

↻ REPEAT the set for a total of three rounds
◷ REST 1:00 before set C

 SET C

DEEP SQUAT	
15x	P102

ARCHER PULL-UP	
10x	P108

DRAGON WALK	
0:45	P128

↻ REPEAT the set for a total of three rounds
◷ REST 1:00 before set D

SET D

PIGEON PEEL AND BUTTERFLY PEEL	
15x each	P122

INVERTED BODWEIGHT ROW	
10x	P054

MOUNTAIN CLIMBER	
0:45	P043

↻ REPEAT the set for a total of three rounds
◷ REST 1:00

CORE POWER
Perform all exercises in order and rest for 30 seconds. Complete four rounds.

HANGING LEG RAISE	
10x	P110

HOLLOW BODY HOLD	
0:30	P113

HANGING REVERSE CURL	
10x	P116

BACK BRIDGE	
0:30	P120

◷ REST 0:30
↻ REPEAT Core Power for a total of four rounds

SUPER CIRCUIT PER-4-MANCE

Combining HIIT with compound strength training, this four-set workout decreases body fat percentage, increases lean muscle mass, boosts athletic performance, and improves agility.

High intensity interval training (HIIT), used in sets A and C, should elevate your heart rate to 80–90 per cent of its maximum. You should be out of breath and unable to hold a conversation. HIIT has been proven to boost muscle-producing hormones such as HGH and testosterone.

Complete all sets in order (A–D) for the prescribed number of rounds. Rest for one minute between each set.

SET A

DEEP SQUAT	
work 0:20, rest 0:10	**P**102

SINGLE-LEG BURPEE – LEFT	
work 0:20, rest 0:10	**P**134

SINGLE-LEG BURPEE – RIGHT	
work 0:20, rest 0:10	**P**134

SKATER JUMP	
work 0:20, rest 0:10	**P**130

↻ REPEAT set A for a total of four rounds
🕐 REST 1:00 before set B

SET B

FRONT LUNGE	
15x	**P**104

ALTERNATING CROSS-OVER LUNGE	
15x	**P**106

BULGARIAN SPLIT SQUAT	
15x	**P**124

PIGEON PEEL AND BUTTERFLY PEEL	
15x each	**P**122

🕐 REST 1:00
↻ REPEAT set B for a total of two rounds
🕐 REST 1:00 before set C

SET C

1–2 PUSH	
work 0:20, rest 0:10	**P**126

HANGING LEG RAISE	
work 0:20, rest 0:10	**P**110

BACKWARDS PRESS-UP	
work 0:20, rest 0:10	**P**132

HANGING REVERSE CURL	
work 0:20, rest 0:10	**P**116

↻ REPEAT set C for a total of four rounds
🕐 REST 1:00 before set D

SET D

ARCHER PULL-UP	
10x	**P**108

STOP-AND-GO PRESS-UP	
10x	**P**138

INVERTED BODYWEIGHT ROW	
10x	**P**054

FOREARM PRESS-UP	
10x	**P**112

🕐 REST 1:00
↻ REPEAT set D for a total of two rounds
🕐 REST 1:00

TRI-SET

Each set in this workout is composed of three complementary exercises with lower body versus upper body, or push offsetting pull, to maximize the efficiency of the workout. This ensures you have enough left in the tank to complete each muscle-building, body-sculpting rep with great form.

ARCHER PULL-UP

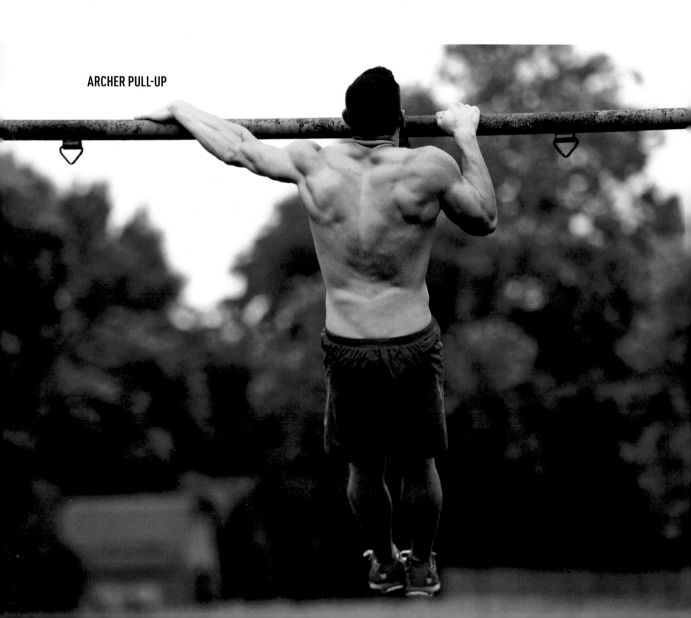

Perform each set for five rounds, subtracting two reps per round (pyramid format). Complete all five rounds of a set before resting one minute and moving on to the next set.

SET A

DEEP SQUAT

| 10x, 8x, 6x, 4x, 2x | P102 |

ARCHER PULL-UP

| 10x, 8x, 6x, 4x, 2x | P108 |

PIKE PRESS-UP TO PRESS-UP

| 10x, 8x, 6x, 4x, 2x | P140 |

↻ REPEAT for five rounds in pyramid format
🕐 REST 1:00 before set B

SET B

FRONT LUNGE

| 10x, 8x, 6x, 4x, 2x | P104 |

PIGEON PEEL AND BUTTERFLY PEEL

| 10x, 8x, 6x, 4x, 2x each | P122 |

STOP-AND-GO PRESS-UP

| 10x, 8x, 6x, 4x, 2x | P138 |

↻ REPEAT for five rounds in pyramid format
🕐 REST 1:00 before set C

SET C

ALTERNATING CROSS-OVER LUNGE

| 10x, 8x, 6x, 4x, 2x | P106 |

FOREARM PRESS-UP

| 10x, 8x, 6x, 4x, 2x | P112 |

CHIN-UP

| 10x, 8x, 6x, 4x, 2x | P050 |

↻ REPEAT for five rounds in pyramid format
🕐 REST 1:00 before set D

SET D

BULGARIAN SPLIT SQUAT

| 10x, 8x, 6x, 4x, 2x each side | P124 |

SKATER JUMP

| 10x, 8x, 6x, 4x, 2x each side | P130 |

FROG HOLD

| 0:45 | P110 |

↻ REPEAT for five rounds in pyramid format
🕐 REST 1:00

> If you're having a hard time recovering between sets, increase the rest period to two minutes and make the exercises easier as needed.

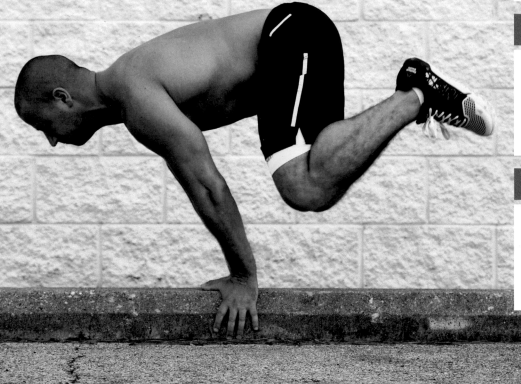

PROGRAMME

The workouts in weeks 1 and 3 repeat, as do the ones for weeks 2 and 4. You will have six days of work and one of rest. It's best to perform the workouts Monday to Saturday and rest on Sunday, but if your schedule doesn't permit that, it's okay to schedule your rest day as needed. You should avoid switching workouts within the programme to rest the muscle groups properly.

WEEK 1

WEEK 2

WEEK 3

WEEK 4

DAY **01**	DAY **02**	DAY **03**	DAY **04**	DAY **05**	DAY **06**
• HERCULES WORKOUT • FINISHER	• CRAZY 8s • CORE POWER	• YUE FEI WORKOUT • FINISHER	• PUSH-PULL PAIRS • RIP IT	• HANNIBAL WORKOUT • FINISHER	• SUPER CIRCUIT FANTASTIC FOUR

DAY **08**	DAY **09**	DAY **10**	DAY **11**	DAY **12**	DAY **13**
• LEGENDARY LEGS	• TRI-PHASE • CORE POWER	• FIRE	• ALL-IN • RIP IT	• TRI-SET	• SUPER CIRCUIT PER-4-MANCE

DAY **15**	DAY **16**	DAY **17**	DAY **18**	DAY **19**	DAY **20**
• HERCULES WORKOUT • FINISHER	• CRAZY 8s • CORE POWER	• YUE FEI WORKOUT • FINISHER	• PUSH-PULL PAIRS • RIP IT	• HANNIBAL WORKOUT • FINISHER	• SUPER CIRCUIT FANTASTIC FOUR

DAY **22**	DAY **23**	DAY **24**	DAY **25**	DAY **26**	DAY **27**
• LEGENDARY LEGS	• TRI-PHASE • RIP IT	• FIRE	• ALL-IN • RIP IT	• TRI-SET	• SUPER CIRCUIT PER-4-MANCE

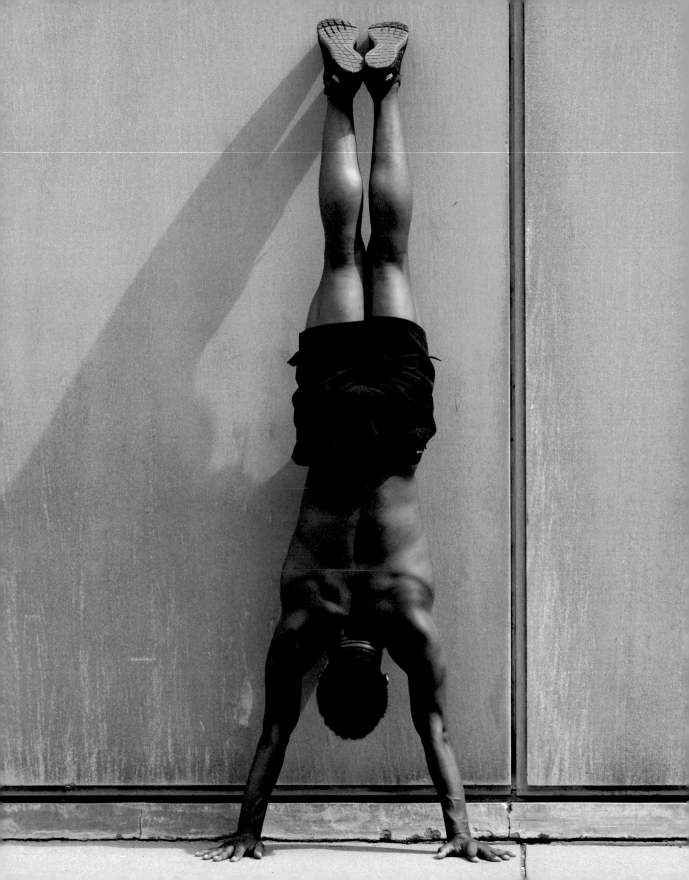

LEVEL 3

Level 3 introduces explosive power through plyometrics, forming exercises from previous levels into dynamic and mobile combinations. This level increases the demands upon your body with single-limb, unilateral exercises for greater weight loss and definition.

HANDSTAND WALK

Handstands are an excellent way to build strong, stable shoulders and a bulletproof core. The handstand walk provides all these benefits, and its ability to improve balance will give you confidence.

MORE DIFFICULT

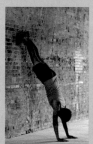

Modify stability: Omit step 4. Instead, in step 3, bring your legs parallel to the floor and place your feet on the wall in an L-stand. This extends your body from the wall and transfers weight into the upper body.

LESS DIFFICULT

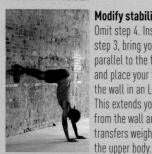

Modify body angle: In step 4, decrease the space between your hands and the wall. Not extending the body as far from the wall will decrease the load on your core.

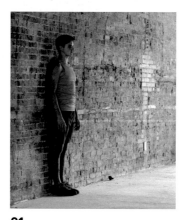

01 Stand facing away from a wall with your heels placed at the base of it.

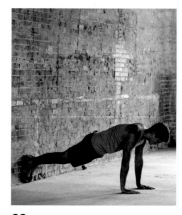

02 Lower into a plank position with your weight evenly distributed between hands and toes.

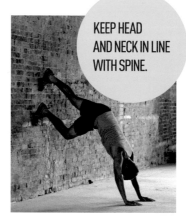

KEEP HEAD AND NECK IN LINE WITH SPINE.

03 Slowly walk your feet up the wall, moving your hands closer to it as you climb with your feet. Keep arms straight.

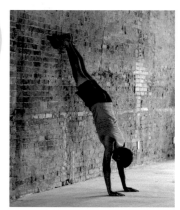

04 Try to get as close to the wall as possible in a handstand position.

Handstand walks prepare your arms and shoulders to bear your bodyweight when inverted in a handstand, and train your body to stay rigid and stable.

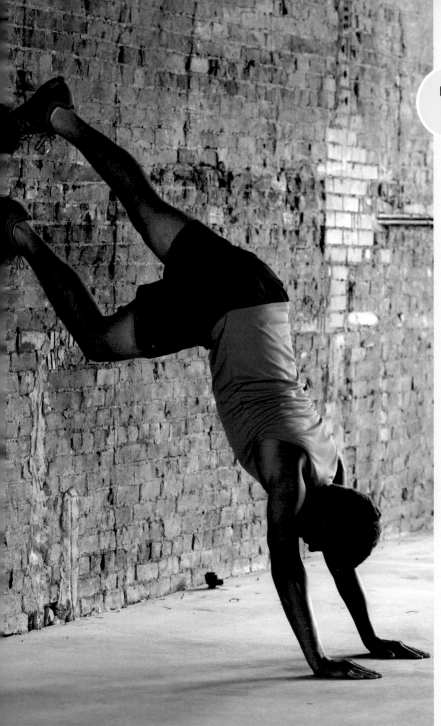

Try this ...

Add a press-up to the handstand or the L-stand (which is the More Difficult version on page 162).

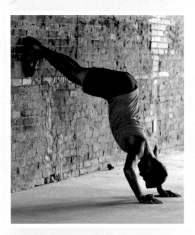

L-STAND PRESS-UP

When in the L-stand described in More Difficult, bend the elbows and lower the crown of the head to the floor, then press through the palms and straighten your arms.

05 Reverse step 3 by slowly walking your hands away from the wall and lowering your feet to the floor to return to the plank position.

HOLLOW BODY ROCKER

While the motion is only small, adding a "rock" to the hollow body position will challenge your core like never before.

MORE DIFFICULT

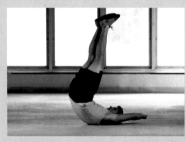

Modify range of motion: In step 3, rock until your hips lift off of the floor to increase the range of motion and generate greater force for your core to control.

LESS DIFFICULT

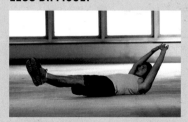

Modify speed: Omit step 3. Instead, hold the position in step 2, building strength and preparing to add motion later.

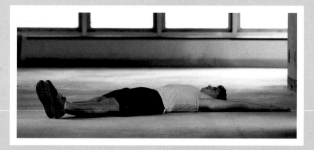

01 Lie on your back with arms and legs extended, pull your belly button in towards the floor, and tuck your pelvis to connect your lower back to the floor.

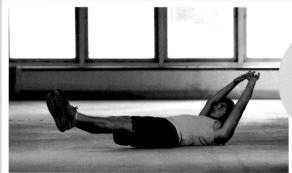

RETAIN A POSTERIOR TILT IN THE PELVIS.

02 Slowly raise your legs, shoulders, and head off of the floor. Hold this "hollow" curved position as you procced to the next step.

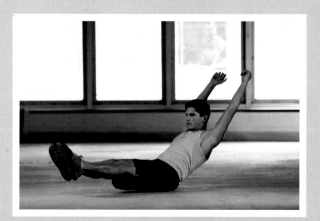

03 Gently rock back and forth on the curve of your lower back. Don't swing your arms or legs. Rock for the duration of the exercise.

SQUAT JUMP

A metabolic-boosting super exercise, the squat jump takes every ounce of energy and coordination while making quads, glutes, and hamstrings all beg for mercy.

MORE DIFFICULT

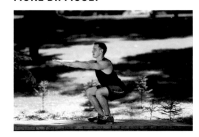

Modify speed: Hold the squat position in step 2 for a count of four upon landing. This removes momentum and creates an isolation hold at its deepest point.

LESS DIFFICULT

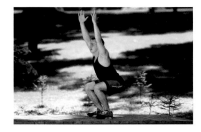

Modify range of motion: Omit steps 3 and 4. Change step 2, lifting arms overhead, and focus on the depth of the squat.

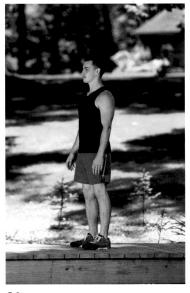

01 Stand tall with your feet shoulder-width apart and your toes pointing forwards.

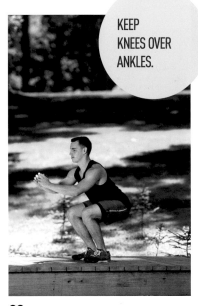

KEEP KNEES OVER ANKLES.

02 With your bodyweight in your heels, inhale as you bend at the knee and lower your body as if about to sit in a chair.

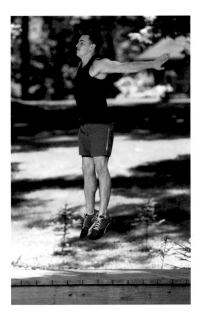

03 Engage your core and exhale as you jump up, pushing through the heels.

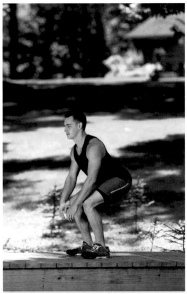

04 Land as softly and silently as possible, bending at the ankles, knees, and hips to decelerate the body.

PISTOL SQUAT

Pistol squats are incredibly difficult but highly effective. They build monstrously strong legs whilst improving balance and mobility.

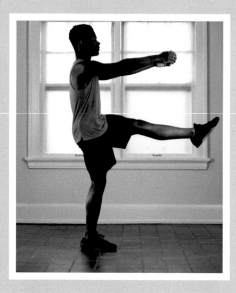

01 Stand with arms extended in front. Balance on one leg with the opposite leg extended straight forwards as high as possible.

MORE DIFFICULT

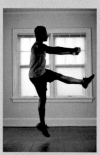

Modify range of motion: As you stand up after step 3, add a little hop. This plyometric motion generates power and makes you decelerate your body using glutes and hamstrings.

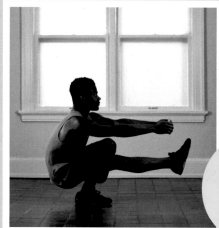

02 Bend the stabilizing leg and lower into as deep a squat as possible while keeping the opposite leg elevated. The supporting knee should point in the same direction as the foot.

DON'T LET BENDING KNEE ROTATE IN OR OUT.

LESS DIFFICULT

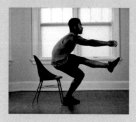

Modify range of motion: With a bench or similar prop behind you, lower only that far in step 2 to build confidence.

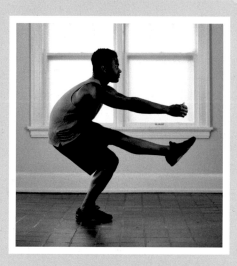

03 Press through the heel of the bent leg, straighten it, and raise the body to the original position until the supporting leg is straight. Complete all reps for one side, then repeat all steps using the other leg.

PLANCHE

The planche is a fundamental gymnastics skill in which the body is held parallel to the floor supported only by hands and arms, with the feet raised.

MORE DIFFICULT

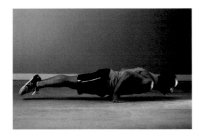

Modify range of motion: Perform press-ups while holding the planche in step 2 to provide a dynamic balance challenge for the core.

LESS DIFFICULT

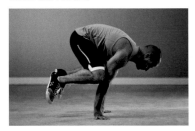

Modify stability: In step 2, tuck the knees to shorten the body, increase balance, and build strength to straighten the legs later.

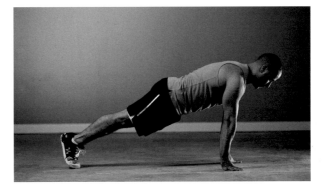

01 Start in a plank position with weight distributed between the hands and toes. Lean your body forwards until the shoulders are in front of the wrists.

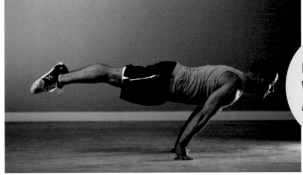

KEEP HIPS LEVEL WITH SHOULDERS AND GLUTES.

02 Inhale and transfer your full weight into your arms, elevating your feet. Hold this "floating" position with hips and shoulders level.

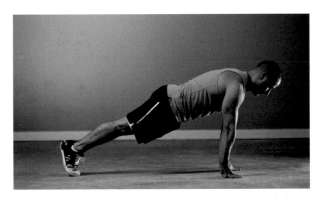

03 Carefully lower your feet and transfer your weight until it's evenly distributed between hands and toes.

ONE-ARM CHIN-UP

One-arm chin-ups are a super exercise requiring greater strength, coordination, and balance than the standard chin-up found in Level 1.

MORE DIFFICULT

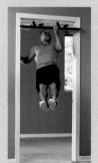

Modify speed: In step 3, lower slowly over a count of four, creating an eccentric muscle contraction to build incredible strength and power.

LESS DIFFICULT

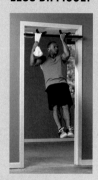

Modify points of contact: Use a towel around the bar to assist the non-working arm. The towel provides stability and can be pulled with that arm to create leverage.

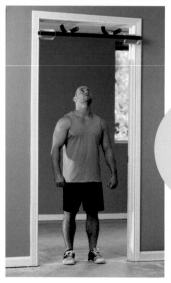

01 Stand directly under your pull-up bar.

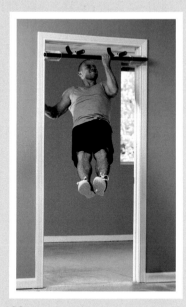

A STRONG GRIP CONTRACTS THE UPPER-BODY MUSCLES.

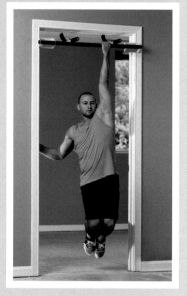

02 Grab the bar with a one-arm underhand grip (palm facing you) and hang with a straight arm.

03 Pull yourself up until your chin is above the bar, and pause. Lower yourself down with control.

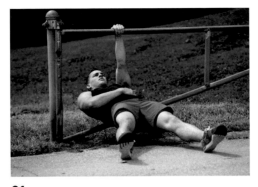

01 Lie on your back directly under the bar. Grab the bar with one hand in an overhand grip (palm facing away), hand outside the shoulder.

ONE-ARM INVERTED ROW

This exercise balances the muscles used in press-ups, making it essential for back strength, shoulder stability, and injury prevention.

MORE DIFFICULT

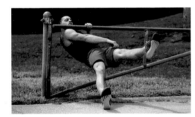

Modify stability and range of motion: In all steps, elevating a foot on a prop decreases leverage in the legs, so you pull more weight and challenge balance and strength.

LESS DIFFICULT

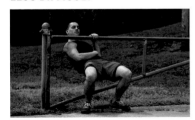

Modify stability and points of contact: In all steps, bend one or both legs to create leverage so you can focus on form.

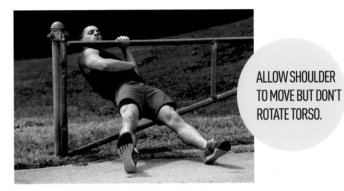

ALLOW SHOULDER TO MOVE BUT DON'T ROTATE TORSO.

02 Pull yourself up until your chest touches the bar, and pause.

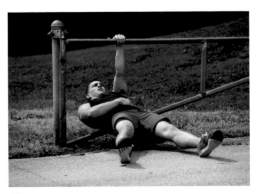

03 Lower yourself down with control.

FRONT LEVER

The front lever is a fundamental gymnastics strength hold that develops the core and upper body muscles.

MORE DIFFICULT

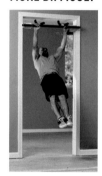

Modify range of motion: Remove the tuck in step 2 and elevate from dead hang to front lever, shifting your weight and forcing the core and lats to work overtime to keep you elevated.

LESS DIFFICULT

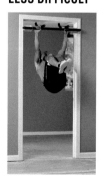

Modify range of motion: Omit step 3. Instead, tuck the knees into a tabletop position and hold to decrease your leverage and the force working against gravity.

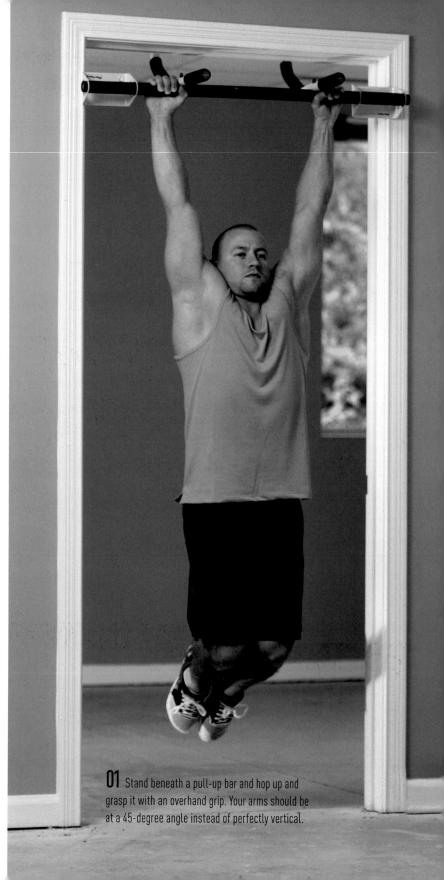

01 Stand beneath a pull-up bar and hop up and grasp it with an overhand grip. Your arms should be at a 45-degree angle instead of perfectly vertical.

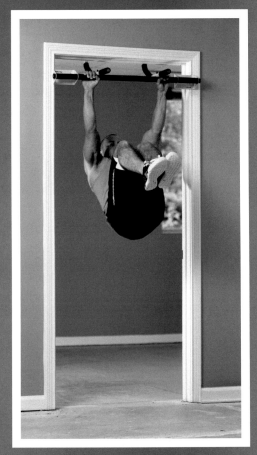

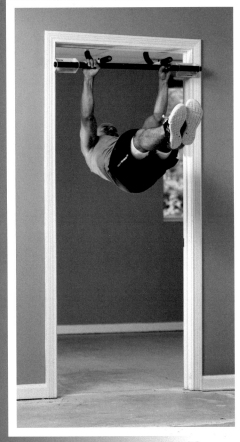

02 Tuck knees into chest and rock back until your body hangs in a ball-like position.

03 Straighten legs, press through straight arms to engage the lats, and form a straight line from shoulders to toes. Hold this position for the duration of the exercise.

ROTATE HANDS SLIGHTLY SO PALMS FACE DOWN.

The front lever is a popular gymnastics hold because it's an impressive display of strength that helps develop a strong core and powerful pulling muscles.

SINGLE-LEG REVERSE BRIDGE

Back bridges are one of the best back exercises for building total body strength and flexibility.

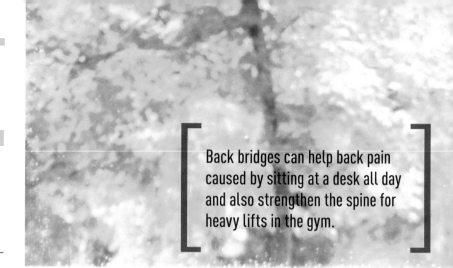

[Back bridges can help back pain caused by sitting at a desk all day and also strengthen the spine for heavy lifts in the gym.]

MORE DIFFICULT

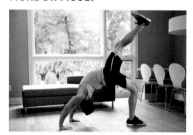

Modify range of motion: In step 2, add an extra half rep by lowering halfway and then re-engaging the core and glutes to lift back up.

LESS DIFFICULT

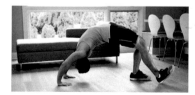

Modify points of contact: Instead of elevating the leg vertically in step 2, extend it horizontally and rest the heel on the floor to provide balance and stability.

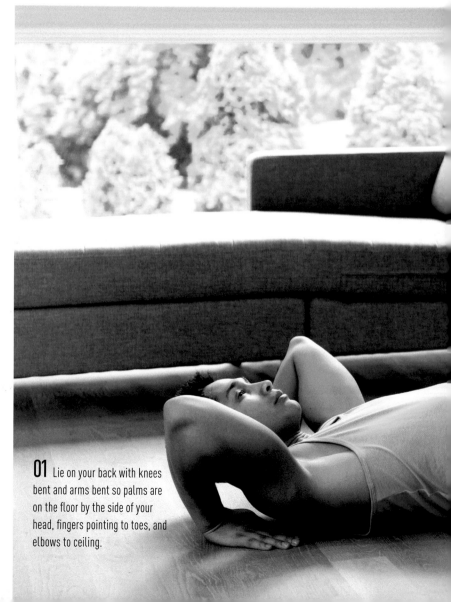

01 Lie on your back with knees bent and arms bent so palms are on the floor by the side of your head, fingers pointing to toes, and elbows to ceiling.

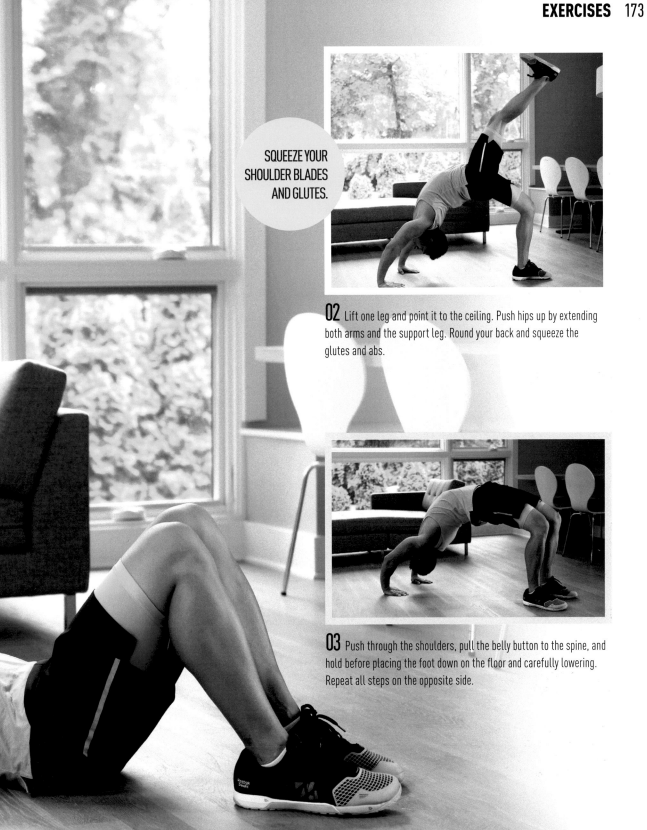

SQUEEZE YOUR
SHOULDER BLADES
AND GLUTES.

02 Lift one leg and point it to the ceiling. Push hips up by extending both arms and the support leg. Round your back and squeeze the glutes and abs.

03 Push through the shoulders, pull the belly button to the spine, and hold before placing the foot down on the floor and carefully lowering. Repeat all steps on the opposite side.

NEO ROW

I can't promise you'll be able to dodge bullets after this exercise, but you will build a bulletproof back, shoulders, and core; increase athletic performance; and feel like an action hero.

MORE DIFFICULT

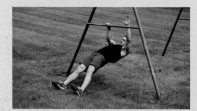

Modify speed: In step 3, lower from the bar slowly over a count of four to create a strength-building eccentric muscle contraction.

LESS DIFFICULT

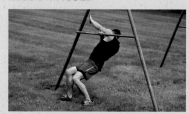

Modify points of contact: For all steps, bend one or both legs to decrease the amount of bodyweight working against gravity and increase stability. Focus on your form.

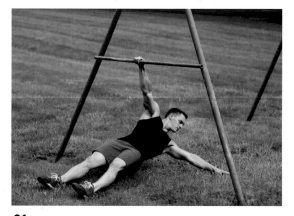

01 Lie on your back under the bar. Grab it overhand with one hand held wider than the shoulder. Allow the non-working arm and shoulder to rotate towards the ground, but keep hips square.

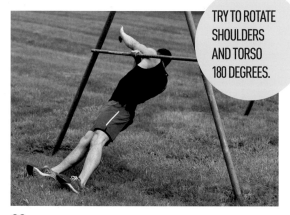

TRY TO ROTATE SHOULDERS AND TORSO 180 DEGREES.

02 Pull yourself towards the bar and take the non-pulling arm across the body, rotating shoulders and reaching to the outside of the arm on the bar. Pause and hold for a second.

Don't use momentum to throw your arm up and across your body. Instead, control the motion and rotate your core.

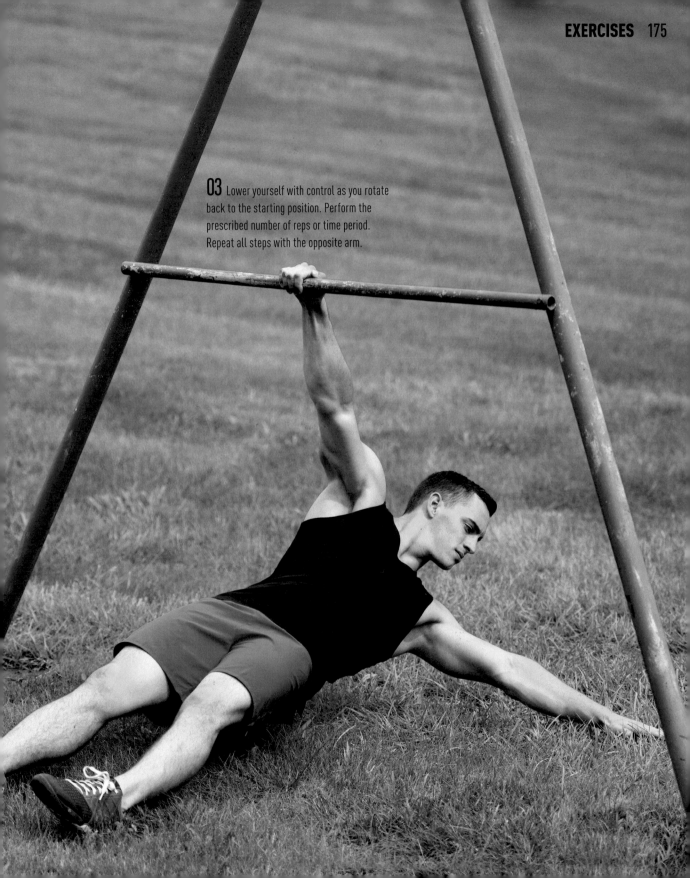

03 Lower yourself with control as you rotate back to the starting position. Perform the prescribed number of reps or time period. Repeat all steps with the opposite arm.

PANCAKE PRESS-UP

This "double-stacks" the perfect compound exercise – extending the arms overhead to decrease upper body leverage, and requiring incredible core strength.

MORE DIFFICULT

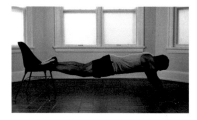

Modify body angle: Elevate your feet on a box or bench to decline your body, shifting a greater proportion of bodyweight into the upper body.

LESS DIFFICULT

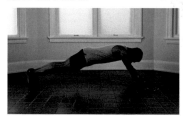

Modify speed: Hold an extended plank for a time to build strength and confidence as you work up to performing the pancake press-up.

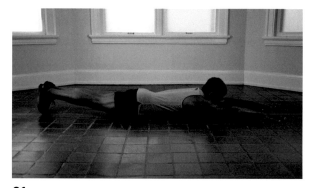

01 Lie face-down on the floor, arms extended overhead, and legs extended but toes curled under on the floor. Inhale.

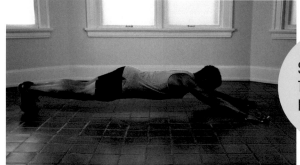

02 On the exhale, press down into the floor through the palms, using full extension of the arms for leverage and lifting the body off the floor. Hold for a count of two.

SPREAD FINGER TIPS WIDE FOR MORE STABILITY.

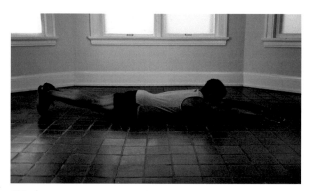

03 Inhale and slowly lower the body to the floor. Repeat steps 2 and 3 for the duration of the exercise.

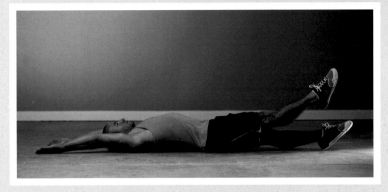

FLUTTER UP

This advanced core exercise engages the abdominals, erector spinae, and hip flexors as you fight to elevate the upper and lower body in unison.

01 Lie on your back with arms and legs extended, and with one leg approximately 30cm (12in) higher than the other.

MORE DIFFICULT

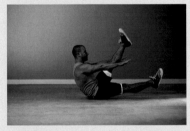

Modify range of motion: In steps 2 and 3, add a half rep after each full rep by lowering halfway and raising back up, performing 50 per cent more work and punishing your core.

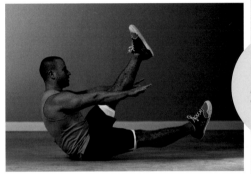

KEEP NECK SOFT AND HEAD ALIGNED WITH SPINE.

02 Switch the feet in increments of 30cm (12in) as you simultaneously lift the torso and legs to form a V, with the arms reaching towards the fluttering toes.

LESS DIFFICULT

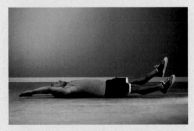

Modify range of motion: Keep your upper body still and only flutter your legs. Focus on proper form in your posterior pelvic tilt.

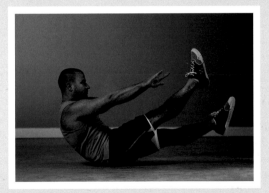

03 Continue to flutter the legs as you slowly lower your torso back to the floor. Repeat steps 2 and 3 for the duration of the exercise.

BURPEE TO PULL-UP

This combines two insanely effective exercises into one compound total-body strength and cardiovascular powerhouse.

MORE DIFFICULT

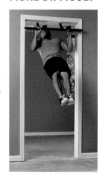

Modify speed: In step 7, lower over a count of four. This requires a strength-building, gravity-defying, eccentric muscle contraction.

LESS DIFFICULT

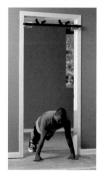

Modify range of motion: Eliminate the press-up in step 2 to perform a squat thrust to chin-up instead. This decreases work but lets you move faster and improves cardiovascular fitness.

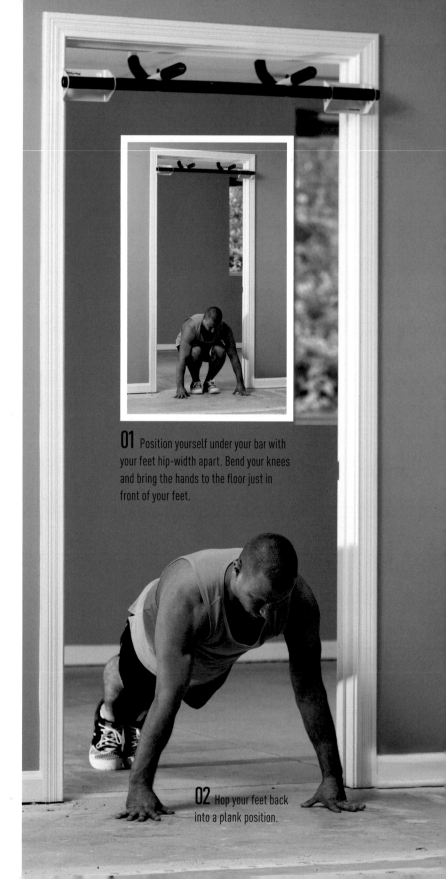

01 Position yourself under your bar with your feet hip-width apart. Bend your knees and bring the hands to the floor just in front of your feet.

02 Hop your feet back into a plank position.

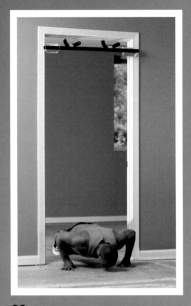

03 Perform one press-up with your core engaged.

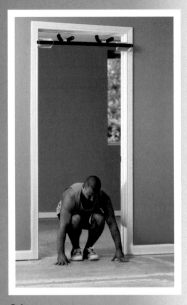

04 Jump to bring your feet back to your hands, shifting your weight to the heels and lifting your chest.

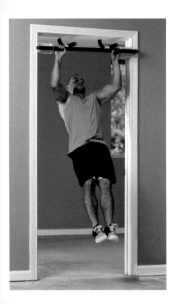

05 Jump from the crouched position and reach hands overhead to grasp the bar in an overhand grip with hands wider than shoulders.

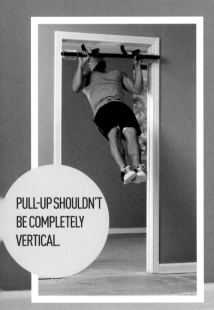

PULL-UP SHOULDN'T BE COMPLETELY VERTICAL.

06 Pull yourself up until your chin is above the bar. Touch your chest to the bar with a slightly backwards lean to the body.

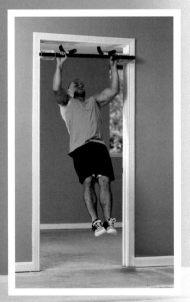

07 Lower yourself to the floor by straightening the arms. Make sure to do this with control, as it will build strength.

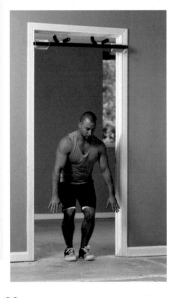

08 Let go of the bar, landing softly with a slight bend at your knees, hips, and ankles.

PLYOMETRIC INVERTED ROW

In plyometrics, the muscles exert maximum force in short time intervals, with the goal of adding both speed and power to an exercise.

MORE DIFFICULT

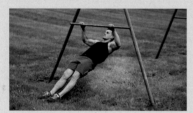

Modify speed: In step 3, lower slowly over four seconds to add a strength-building eccentric muscle contraction.

LESS DIFFICULT

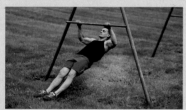

Modify stability and points of contact: Don't let go of the bar in step 2. Instead, perform an inverted bodyweight row, pulling as aggressively as possible on the way up.

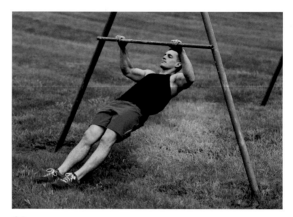

01 Lie on your back directly under the bar. Grab the bar with an overhand grip, hands wider than your shoulders.

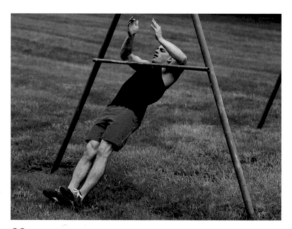

02 Pull yourself up aggressively and try to "jump" your chest to the bar while you let go and extend your arms past the bar.

[Start small with the "jump". Begin by lightly letting go of the bar, and build to a full extension or clap above the bar.]

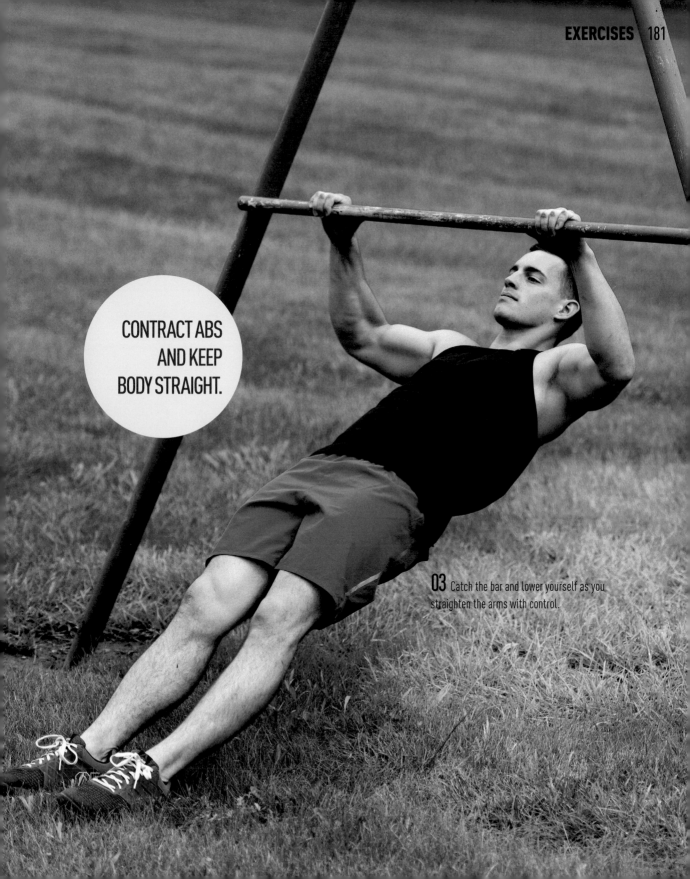

CONTRACT ABS
AND KEEP
BODY STRAIGHT.

03 Catch the bar and lower yourself as you
straighten the arms with control.

PEDAL

The pedal, or jump lunge, will make your heart rate skyrocket and your lower body scream. This quad and glute killer requires balance, coordination, and more than a little determination.

MORE DIFFICULT

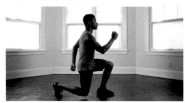

Modify speed: Upon landing in step 3, hold for a count of four to add a strength-building isolation hold and remove momentum.

LESS DIFFICULT

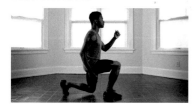

Modify range of motion: Remove the jump in step 3; instead perform a back lunge, alternating legs and focusing on depth of motion.

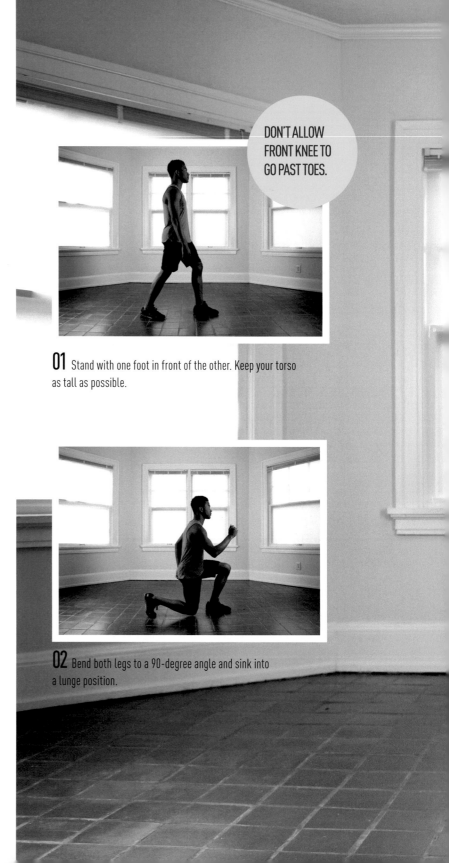

DON'T ALLOW FRONT KNEE TO GO PAST TOES.

01 Stand with one foot in front of the other. Keep your torso as tall as possible.

02 Bend both legs to a 90-degree angle and sink into a lunge position.

Try this ...

Increase the depth of the exercise and challenge the inner thighs, hips, and glutes.

03 Jump with enough force to propel both feet from the floor. While in the air, scissor-switch your feet. Land in a lunge position with the opposite foot in front.

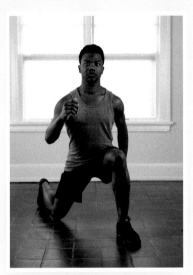

STAGGERED PEDAL
In step 2, widen your stance, opening the legs to just past shoulder width.

Pay attention to the impact during the landing. Land as softly as possible so the force of the deceleration is distributed between knee, hip, and ankle joints.

L-SIT CHIN-UP

This exercise builds on the classic chin-up by adding a challenging isolation hold for hip flexors, quads, and abdominals.

MORE DIFFICULT

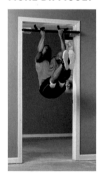

Modify speed: In step 3, lower from the chin-up slowly over a count of four to add a strength-building eccentric muscle contraction.

LESS DIFFICULT

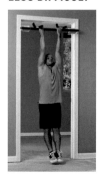

Modify range of motion: Omit steps 3 and 4 to simply hang from the bar and perform leg raises, which will strengthen your grip. This allows you to focus on building core strength.

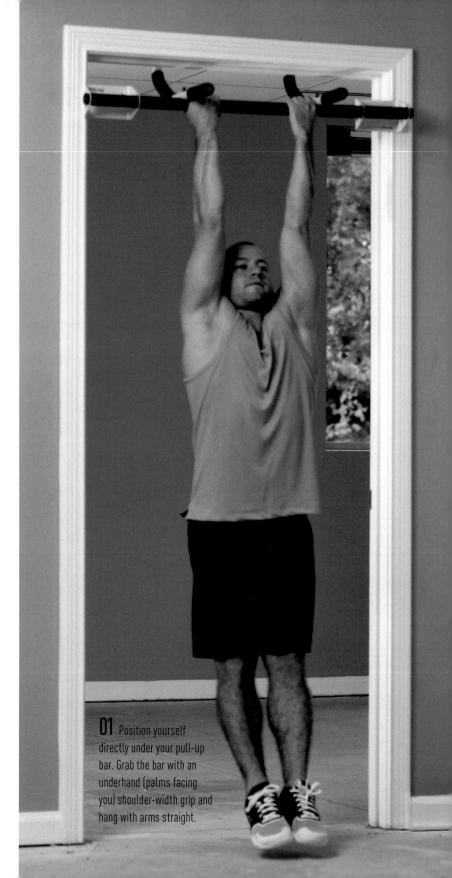

01 Position yourself directly under your pull-up bar. Grab the bar with an underhand (palms facing you) shoulder-width grip and hang with arms straight.

When you perform an L-sit for the first time, you may struggle to fully straighten your legs. Weakness in the quads or abdominals, or even lack of flexibility in the hamstrings, can make quads feel about to cramp.

LIFT LEGS UNTIL TOES ARE HIGHER THAN HIPS.

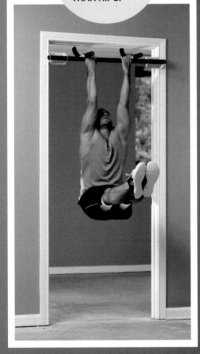

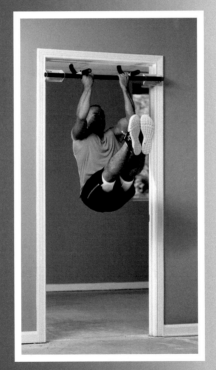

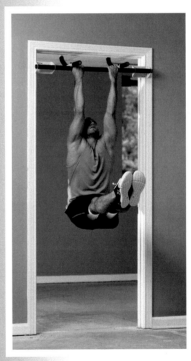

02 Keep legs straight and lift them until they're just beyond parallel to the floor, forming an L with the torso. Toes should be pointed, thighs squeezed together, and knees completely locked.

03 Maintain the L shape and pull yourself up until your chest touches the bar. Squeeze the shoulder blades and pause for a count of two.

04 Lower yourself down by straightening your arms. Don't lower your legs; instead, remain in the L-sit position for the required reps.

SINGLE-LEG PELVIC PEEL

This peel increases strength in the hips, hamstrings, and glutes while simultaneously challenging your balance and proprioception.

MORE DIFFICULT

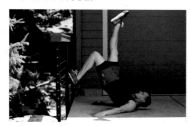

Modify body angle: In all steps, elevate the feet on a prop to shift weight to the hips and core, requiring you to lift hips higher and increasing glute activation.

LESS DIFFICULT

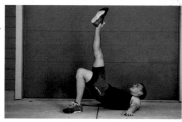

Modify speed: Instead of lifting and lowering, hold the highest point of the exercise to create a strength-building isolation hold.

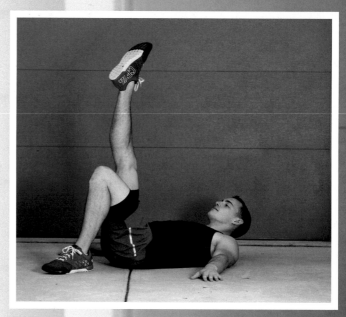

01 Lie flat on your back. Bend one leg and place the foot about 30cm (12in) from your glutes. Elevate the other leg to 90 degrees and point the toes up. Leave arms loose at your sides.

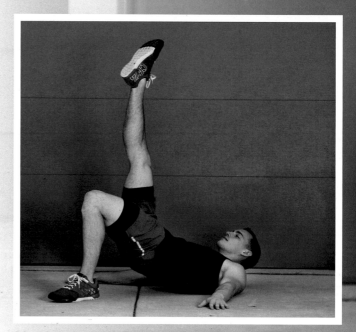

02 Pressing through the sole of the foot on the floor, squeeze the glutes and lift the hips until your body forms a straight line from shoulders to knees. Pause at the top of the motion and hold for one or two seconds.

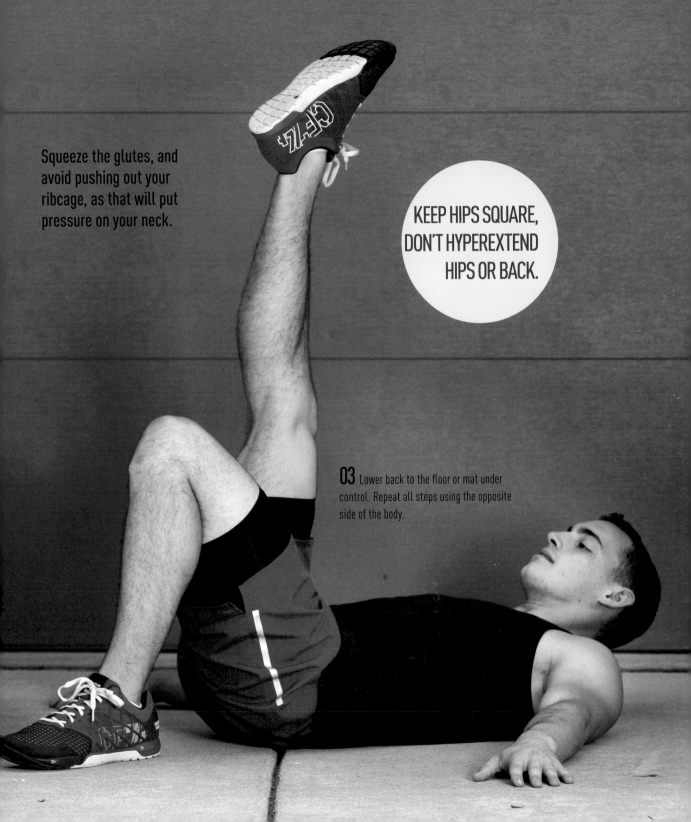

Squeeze the glutes, and avoid pushing out your ribcage, as that will put pressure on your neck.

KEEP HIPS SQUARE, DON'T HYPEREXTEND HIPS OR BACK.

03 Lower back to the floor or mat under control. Repeat all steps using the opposite side of the body.

KNEE TUCK EXTENSION

The knee tuck extension amps up the classic chin-up by adding a challenging isolation hold for hip flexors, quads, and abdominals.

MORE DIFFICULT

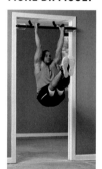

Modify speed: Hold step 3 for a count of four to create a brief isolation hold, which will build strength in the position where you're working against the greatest leverage.

LESS DIFFICULT

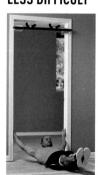

Modify stability: Perform the exercise lying on the floor instead of hanging to increase stability and to build confidence and strength before eventually going to the bar.

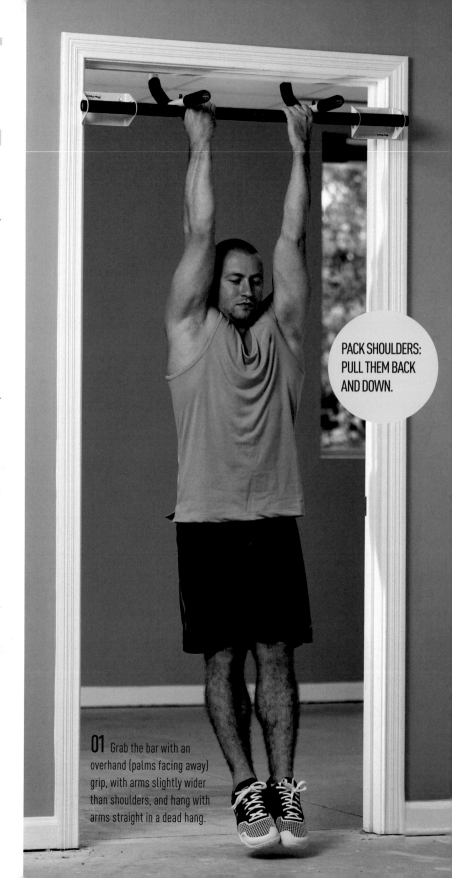

PACK SHOULDERS: PULL THEM BACK AND DOWN.

01 Grab the bar with an overhand (palms facing away) grip, with arms slightly wider than shoulders, and hang with arms straight in a dead hang.

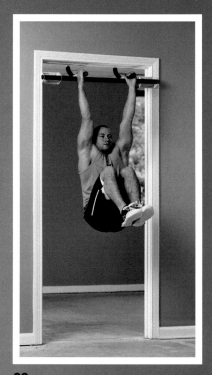

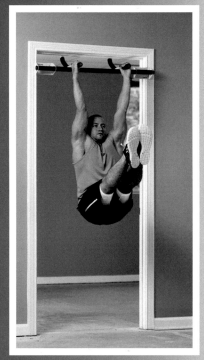

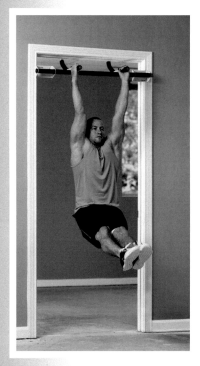

02 Tuck the knees to the chest without causing the body to swing on the bar.

03 Straighten the legs until they're just beyond parallel to the floor, forming an L with the torso. Toes should be pointed, thighs squeezed together, and knees locked.

04 Keep the legs straight and lower them slowly with control until your body forms a straight line, returning to the dead hang position.

Knees up, chin down: The rectus abdominis (six-pack abs) are flexors. If you bring the knees up and tuck the chin slightly, it will encourage the abs to contract.

T-STAND JUMP

Adding an explosive leap to the yoga-inspired T-stand improves athletic performance by forcing you to control your descent and decelerate in a dynamic fashion.

MORE DIFFICULT

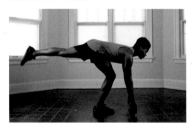

Modify stability: As you land in step 4, single-leg squat for a count of four, removing momentum and creating an isolation hold.

LESS DIFFICULT

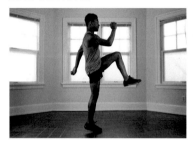

Modify stability: In step 3, bring the knee to the front at hip height, but don't jump. You'll build confidence as you prep to add the jump.

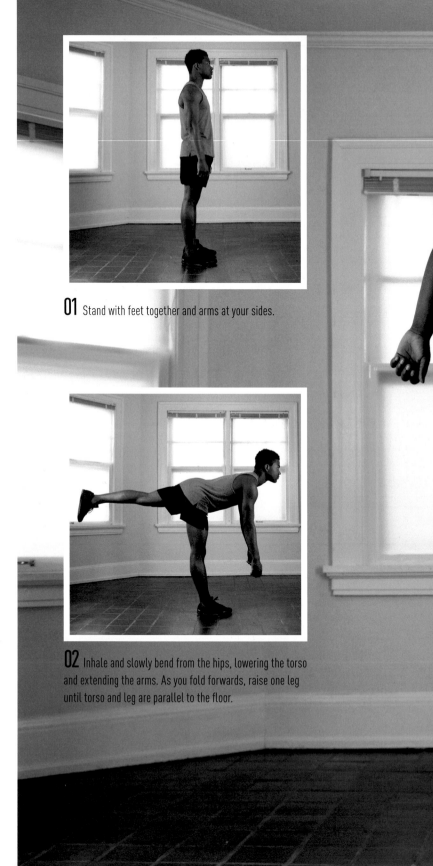

01 Stand with feet together and arms at your sides.

02 Inhale and slowly bend from the hips, lowering the torso and extending the arms. As you fold forwards, raise one leg until torso and leg are parallel to the floor.

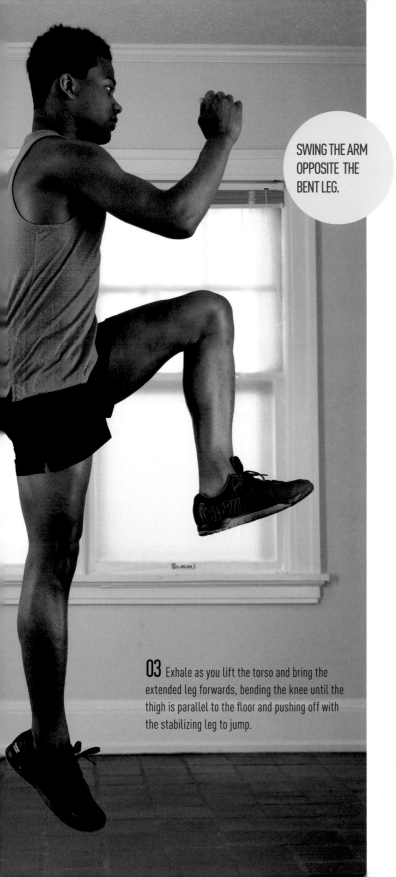

SWING THE ARM
OPPOSITE THE
BENT LEG.

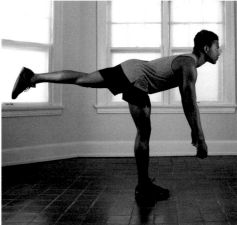

04 Land softly and with control, extending the bent leg to reverse the motion in step 2 and lowering the torso until both are parallel to the floor. Complete all reps on one side of the body, then repeat on the opposite side.

03 Exhale as you lift the torso and bring the extended leg forwards, bending the knee until the thigh is parallel to the floor and pushing off with the stabilizing leg to jump.

If balancing is a challenge, bend deeper at the waist to allow fingertips to touch the floor.

BURPEE TO CHIN-UP

This high-intensity exercise targets the whole body and boosts metabolic conditioning and fat loss. The extreme conditioning it provides also benefits athletic performance.

MORE DIFFICULT

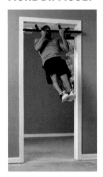

Modify speed: In step 6, lower down over a gravity-defying count of four to add a strength-building eccentric muscle contraction.

LESS DIFFICULT

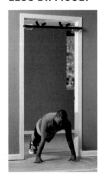

Modify range of motion: Eliminate the press-up in step 2 to perform a squat thrust to chin-up instead. This decreases work but lets you move faster and improves cardiovascular fitness.

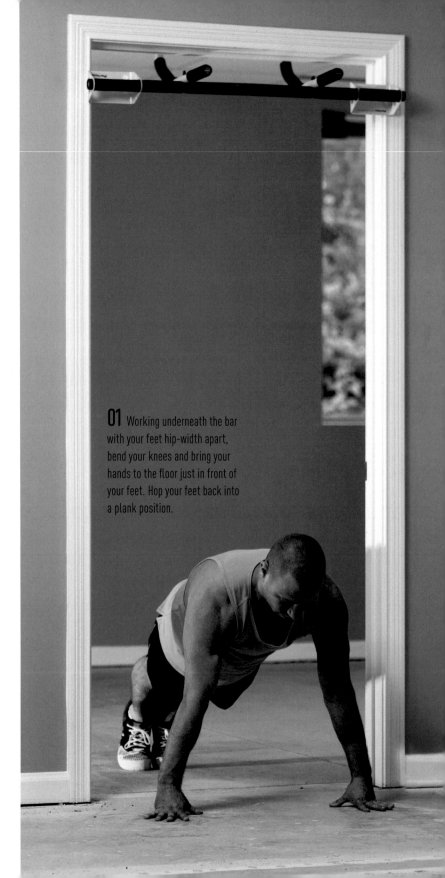

01 Working underneath the bar with your feet hip-width apart, bend your knees and bring your hands to the floor just in front of your feet. Hop your feet back into a plank position.

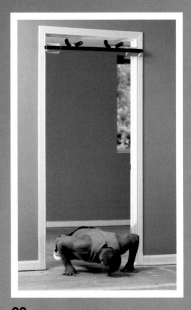

02 Perform one press-up with your core engaged.

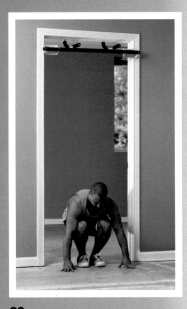

03 Jump to bring your feet back to your hands, shifting your weight into the heels and lifting your chest.

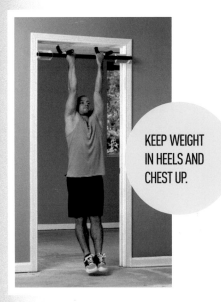

KEEP WEIGHT IN HEELS AND CHEST UP.

04 Jump up and reach hands overhead to grasp the bar in an underhand grip (palms facing towards you).

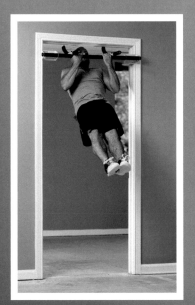

05 Pull yourself up until your chin is above the bar. Squeeze your shoulder blades and try to touch your chest to the bar.

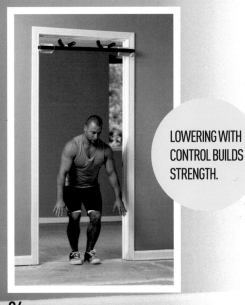

LOWERING WITH CONTROL BUILDS STRENGTH.

06 Lower yourself down by straightening your arms with control. Let go of the bar and land softly with a slight bend at your knees, hips, and ankles.

TUCK JUMP BURPEE

This is an incredible cardiovascular and strength exercise for those feeling superhuman. Explosive plyometrics combined with the total-body Burpee burn fat and improve agility and athletic performance.

MORE DIFFICULT

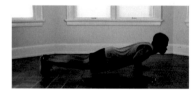

Modify range of motion: In step 3, perform two press-ups, and jump twice in step 5. Twice the effort equals twice the gain.

LESS DIFFICULT

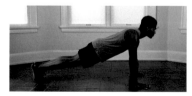

Modify points of contact: Remove the press-up in step 3 and perform a tuck jump squat thrust instead.

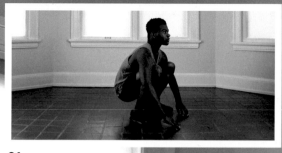

01 With your feet hip-width apart, bend your knees and bring hands to the floor just in front of your feet.

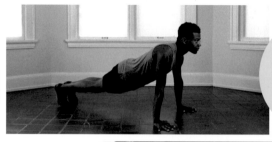

DON'T LET HIPS SAG.

02 Hop your feet back into a plank position with bodyweight evenly distributed between toes and hands, and with the core engaged.

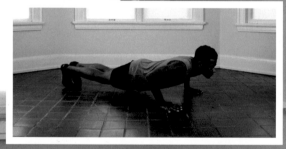

03 Perform one press-up with your core engaged.

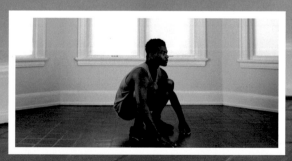

04 Jump your feet back to your hands, shifting your weight into the heels and lifting your chest.

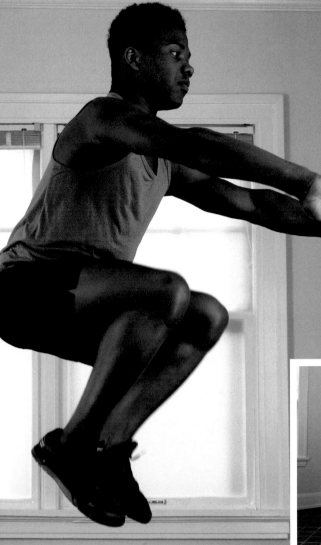

A recent study finds that performing 10 fast-paced repetitions of a Burpee stokes your metabolic furnace as effectively as sprinting for 30 seconds.

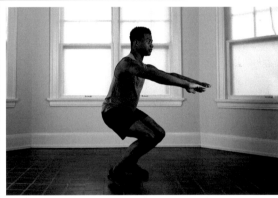

05 Jump up from the crouched position, tucking your knees to your chest.

06 Land softly with a slight bend at your knees, hips, and ankles.

DRAGON FLAG

The dragon flag, created by martial arts legend Bruce Lee, looks insane. It works the entire core and builds incredible strength.

MORE DIFFICULT

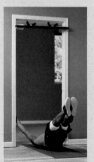

Modify speed: The slower you go, the more time your core has to fight gravity through the eccentric phase of the exercise. This builds incredible core strength.

LESS DIFFICULT

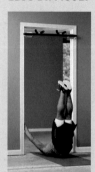

Modify range of motion: Keep your back on the floor in steps 2, 3, and 4, lifting only the hips and legs in those steps. These pikes with a tailbone lift build strength and confidence.

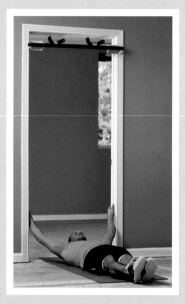

01 Lie on the floor and grab a solid object behind your head with both hands. Create tension throughout your body, starting with traps, lats, and arms.

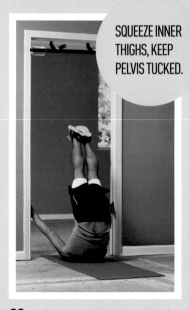

SQUEEZE INNER THIGHS, KEEP PELVIS TUCKED.

02 Keep your core engaged and swing your feet up until your body is almost vertical (shoulder blades should remain on the floor).

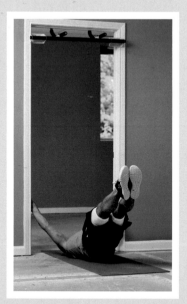

03 Slowly lower your legs under control until they are just above the floor.

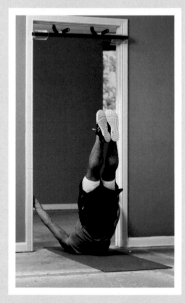

04 Immediately lift the legs back up until you're almost vertical, then slowly lower them under control until they're just above the floor. Repeat steps 2 to 4 for the prescribed time or number of reps.

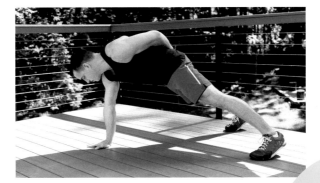

01 Get into press-up position with just one hand on the floor and feet spread wide apart. Tense your entire body and hold your free hand tight against your lower back.

ONE-ARM PRESS-UP

The ultimate show of upper body strength? Some people think so, but the one-arm press-up isn't just for upper body strength because it also engages your core for stability.

MORE DIFFICULT

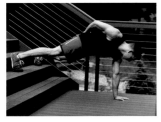

Modify body angle: Elevate feet for all steps to shift a larger percentage of weight into the upper body and work it harder.

LESS DIFFICULT

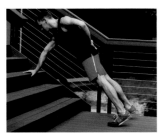

Modify body angle: For all steps, elevate hands, shifting weight to the lower body to work the upper body less.

THE WIDER YOUR FEET, THE EASIER.

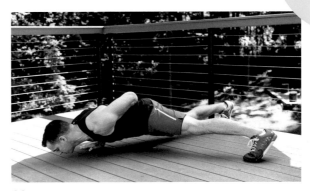

02 Lower your body slowly until your chest nearly touches the ground.

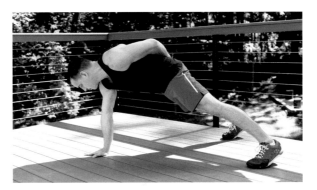

03 Explode up to the starting position, straightening the arm and engaging the core. Perform all prescribed reps on one arm, then repeat with the opposite arm.

SKIN THE CAT

Despite its awful name, this is a great core exercise and also a good stretch for the upper body, especially for achieving full range of motion in the shoulder.

MORE DIFFICULT

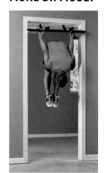

Modify speed: Perform skin the cat as slowly as possible to create dynamic tension and build strength through the eccentric phase of the exercise.

LESS DIFFICULT

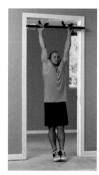

Modify range of motion: Hold a dead hang position for a time to build shoulder and grip strength.

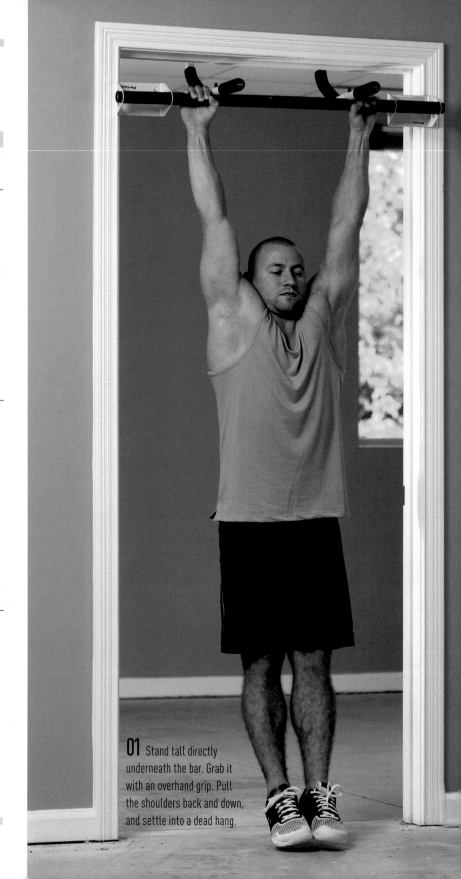

01 Stand tall directly underneath the bar. Grab it with an overhand grip. Pull the shoulders back and down, and settle into a dead hang.

ARMS SHOULD BE
FULLY EXTENDED.

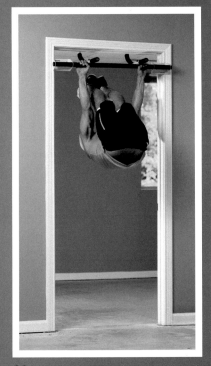

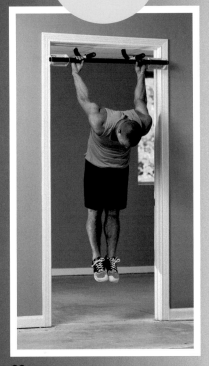

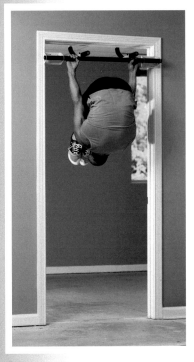

02 Keeping arms and legs straight, point the toes and raise the legs, continuing the movement until the feet pass between the arms and you're in the inverted pike hang position.

03 Continue to pass the feet overhead and down behind you towards the floor (without touching it), rolling your torso so you're in the extended skin-the-cat position.

04 Lift your hips and raise the legs back and over so you're once again in the hanging position from step 1.

Skin the cat stretches and opens up the shoulders to create full range of motion, which helps with press-ups, pull-ups, dips, and front levers.

SQUAT TO L-SIT

This total-body exercise utilizes the lower body and core, and it also engages the hip flexors and triceps isometrically.

MORE DIFFICULT

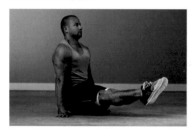

Modify speed: Hold both steps 2 and 5 for a count of four to build strength in the toughest two phases of the exercise.

LESS DIFFICULT

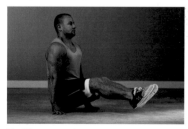

Modify range of motion: In step 5, either extend the legs partially or simply hold them off of the floor in a tucked position.

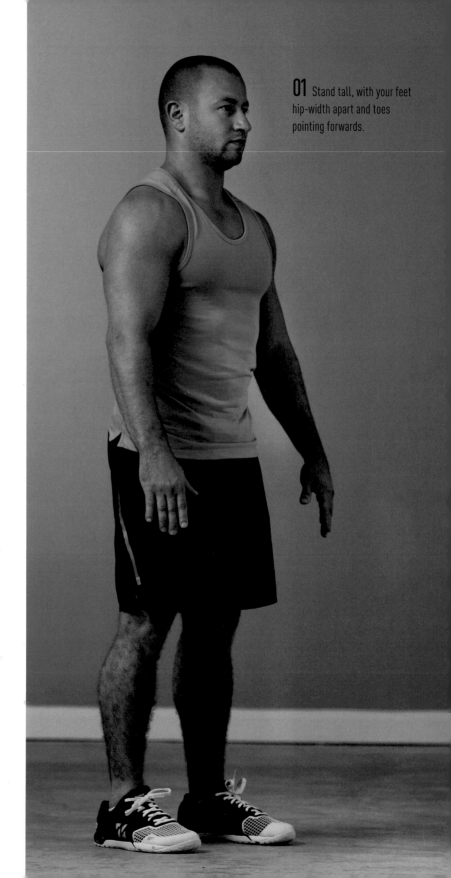

01 Stand tall, with your feet hip-width apart and toes pointing forwards.

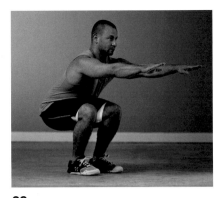

02 Inhale and lower into a deep squat (glutes below knees) as if trying to make glutes touch the back of the calves, arms extended for balance.

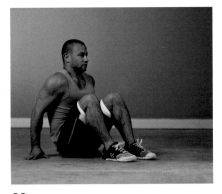

03 Place your hands on the floor slightly behind your hips. Sit, weight shifted back, palms directly under shoulders, fingertips facing forwards.

[
The deeper you can sit into your squat, the easier the transition to L-sit will become.
]

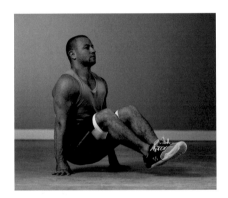

04 Push into the floor with your hands, straighten your arms, and bring your shoulders down in order to lift your butt off of the floor.

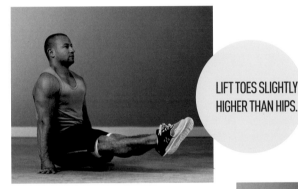

05 Straighten and elevate the legs, squeezing the inner thighs and pointing the toes. Hold this position briefly.

LIFT TOES SLIGHTLY HIGHER THAN HIPS.

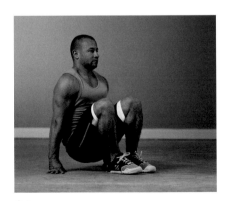

06 Bend and then lower the legs, placing the soles of your feet on the floor.

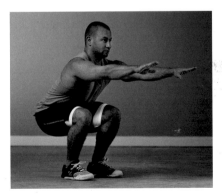

07 Extend your arms in front of you for balance and lift your hips from the floor, rocking yourself slightly forwards into a deep squat.

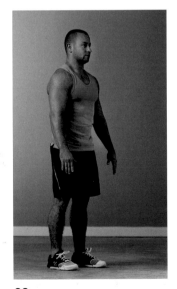

08 Straighten your legs and stand tall, engaging the core, squeezing the glutes, and tucking the hips under.

LEG HELL

It may be short, but this workout certainly isn't sweet! If it's possible to have a "signature" workout, Leg Hell would be mine. Combining lower body exercises from all three levels into a high-intensity circuit with plyometrics might have made Dante Alighieri add one more circle to his vision of the underworld!

SQUAT JUMP

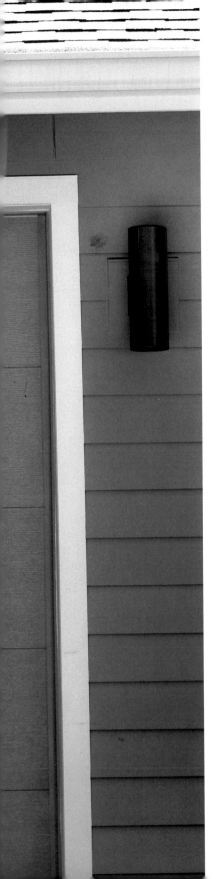

Perform max reps of each exercise for 30 seconds each, then rest for 30 seconds. Complete five rounds.

SQUAT	
0:30	**P**081

BACK LUNGE	
0:30	**P**074

SQUAT JUMP	
0:30	**P**165

PEDAL	
0:30	**P**182

🕐 REST 0:30

↻ REPEAT the set for a total of five rounds

This routine has a 4:1 work-to-rest ratio: work for two minutes, rest for 30 seconds. If that proves too difficult for you to maintain good form, extend the rest periods to one minute to change the ratio to 2:1.

ALEXANDER WORKOUT

The man is called Alexander the Great. If that's not impressive enough to warrant a workout named after him, then consider this: by the age of 33 he had conquered most of the then-known world and he did it all on the front lines. You, too, will meet this workout head on and in an unrelenting fashion if you wish to build strength and lean muscle and dominate on your own personal battlefield, whether that be the gym or the office.

Perform each set for five rounds, subtracting one rep per round where shown (pyramid format). Rest 30 seconds between rounds. Perform all sets and their exercises in order.

 SET A

PISTOL SQUAT	
10x each leg	P166
PANCAKE PRESS-UP	
5x, 4x, 3x, 2x, 1x	P176
BURPEE TO PULL-UP	
5x, 4x, 3x, 2x, 1x	P178

🕐 REST 0:30 after each round of the set
🔁 REPEAT for five rounds in pyramid format

 SET B

PEDAL	
20x each leg	P182
DRAGON FLAG	
5x, 4x, 3x, 2x, 1x	P196
L-SIT CHIN-UP	
5x, 4x, 3x, 2x, 1x	P184

🕐 REST 0:30 after each round of the set
🔁 REPEAT for five rounds in pyramid format

 SET C

SINGLE-LEG PELVIC PEEL	
20x each leg	P186
HANDSTAND WALK	
5x, 4x, 3x, 2x, 1x	P162
PLYOMETRIC INVERTED ROW	
5x, 4x, 3x, 2x, 1x	P180

🕐 REST 0:30 after each round of the set
🔁 REPEAT for five rounds in pyramid format
🔁 REPEAT sets A–C for a total of three rounds

FINISHER
Perform all exercises in order with no rest between rounds.

SQUAT JUMP	
10x	P165
BURPEE TO CHIN-UP	
20x	P192
PEDAL	
30x	P182
MOUNTAIN CLIMBER	
40x	P042

🔁 REPEAT finisher for a total of two rounds

[This is an AsFAP (As Fast As Possible) finisher: but remember that form comes first, and speed second.]

SPARTACUS WORKOUT

A former slave, Spartacus was a heavyweight gladiator (known as a murmillo), which required him to carry a large oblong shield and an 18-inch (46cm) broadsword. He fought his way from the amphitheatres of Rome to lead a 70,000-strong uprising against the mighty Roman Empire. This workout fits his legacy by building rock-solid muscle, challenging balance, and increasing power.

[
If you find this routine too challenging, use the revisions found on the individual exercise pages as substitutes or add a rest period between exercises and/or sets.
]

TABATA-STYLE FINISHER
Push for as many reps as possible in 20 seconds, trying to reach 80–90 per cent of maximum heart rate. Don't rest between rounds. Total exercise time: five minutes.

Perform three full rounds with little or no rest between exercises or rounds.

PISTOL SQUAT	
10x each	P166

ONE-ARM CHIN-UP	
submax*	P168

PANCAKE PRESS-UP	
10x	P176

FRONT LEVER	
0:30	P170

BURPEE TO PULL-UP	
15x	P178

NEO ROW	
10x each side	P174

SQUAT JUMP	
15x	P165

DRAGON FLAG	
10x	P196

↻ REPEAT the set for a total of three rounds

*Submax = 80 per cent of your max number of reps. To calculate your max number of reps, perform the first round to failure (max) and subsequent rounds to 80 per cent of that max number – e.g., max = 10 reps, submax = 8 reps.

TUCK JUMP BURPEE	
work 0:20, rest 0:10	P194

SQUAT JUMP	
work 0:20, rest 0:10	P164

↻ REPEAT Tabata-style finisher for a total of five rounds

PUSH/PULL
POWER

A push/pull split allows you to build muscle and strength without overstressing the body. The efficiency also allows you to train more often.

Perform each set in order. Rest one minute between sets. Complete one to three rounds – if you can't perform every rep with good form, don't progress to the next round.

SET A

STANDARD PRESS-UP	
10x	P048

PULL-UP	
10x	P056

MILITARY PRESS-UP	
10x	P062

CHIN-UP	
10x	P050

🕐 REST 1:00 before set B

SET B

BACKWARDS PRESS-UP	
10x	P132

INVERTED BODYWEIGHT ROW	
10x	P054

STOP-AND-GO PRESS-UP	
10x	P138

CLOSE-GRIP INVERTED ROW	
10x	P052

🕐 REST 1:00 before set C

ARMOUR ABS
Complete exercises in order and rest two minutes. Perform three rounds.

SET C

DOWN DOG PRESS-UP	
10x	P058

L-SIT CHIN-UP	
10x	P184

PLYOMETRIC PRESS-UP	
10x	P136

ARCHER PULL-UP	
10x	P108

🕐 REST 1:00 before set D

SET D

PIKE PRESS-UP TO PRESS-UP	
10x	P140

ONE-ARM INVERTED ROW	
10x each side	P168

PANCAKE PRESS-UP	
10x	P176

PLYOMETRIC INVERTED ROW	
10x	P180

🕐 REST 1:00

🔃 REPEAT sets A–D for one to three rounds

PIKE	
0:30	P052

HANGING LEG RAISE	
0:30	P110

HOLLOW BODY ROCKER	
0:30	P164

KNEE TUCK EXTENSION	
0:30	P188

DRAGON FLAG	
0:30	P196

HANGING REVERSE CURL	
0:30	P116

PLANCHE	
0:30	P167

🕐 REST 2:00

🔃 REPEAT Armour Abs for a total of three rounds

VLAD **WORKOUT**

Very few people in history have cast more terror in the human heart than Vlad the Impaler, or, as he's better known, Dracula. The man who became a legend as the Lord of Darkness was a real person and a great warrior known to drink the blood of his enemies. He was born in 1431 in Transylvania, the central region of modern-day Romania, and ruled for many years, holding the Ottoman Empire at bay. Don't let this workout cast terror in your heart – stay positive and remember that if it doesn't challenge you, it doesn't change you.

Are sore muscles preventing you from progressing or meeting the required reps? Make sure to get adequate pre- and post-workout nutrition, foam roll, and follow the functional exercises. See the Bodyweight Basics section for hints and tips on all those items.

Perform three full rounds with little to no rest between exercises or rounds.

HANDSTAND WALK	
10x	P162

ONE-ARM INVERTED ROW	
10x each side	P169

SQUAT TO L-SIT	
10x	P200

SINGLE-LEG PELVIC PEEL	
10x each side	P186

FRONT LEVER	
0:30	P170

PANCAKE PRESS-UP	
10x	P176

KNEE TUCK EXTENSION	
10x	P188

SKIN THE CAT	
3x with a 10-second hold	P198

↻ REPEAT the set for a total of three rounds

FINISHER
Repeat five times with no rest between rounds. Total exercise time: 10 minutes.

BURPEE TO PULL-UP	
work 0:20, rest 0:10	P178

X-JACK	
work 0:20, rest 0:10	P072

1–2 PUSH	
work 0:20, rest 0:10	P126

BURPEE TO CHIN-UP	
work 0:20, rest 0:10	P192

↻ REPEAT finisher for a total of five rounds

FOUNDATION

A solid foundation creates a strong, balanced, and stable surface that transfers its load to the ground surrounding it. This routine builds the body from the ground up, utilizing some of the biggest muscles in the body to burn calories, build more muscle, and provide a solid footing from which everything else can grow.

Perform the first round to max reps and then aim for 80 per cent of your max reps in the following rounds. For example, if your max is 15 lunges in 30 seconds, aim for 12 lunges while slowing the reps down to meet the 30-second time. This will ensure you can complete all the rounds.

Perform each set in order and rest one minute between sets. Complete three rounds.

SET A

PISTOL SQUAT

10x each side	P166

SINGLE-LEG PELVIC PEEL

10x each side	P186

🕐 **REST 1:00 before set B**

SET B

SQUAT JUMP

20x each side	P165

SINGLE-LEG REVERSE BRIDGE

0:30 each leg	P172

🕐 **REST 1:00 before set C**

SET C

PEDAL

20x	P182

T-STAND JUMP

10x each side	P190

🕐 **REST 1:00**

↻ **REPEAT sets A–C for a total of three rounds**

ARMOUR ABS

Complete exercises in order and rest two minutes. Perform three rounds.

PIKE

0:30	P053

HANGING LEG RAISE

0:30	P110

HOLLOW BODY ROCKER

0:30	P164

KNEE TUCK EXTENSION

0:30	P188

DRAGON FLAG

0:30	P196

HANGING REVERSE CURL

0:30	P116

PLANCHE

0:30	P167

🕐 **REST 2:00**

↻ **REPEAT Armour Abs for a total of three rounds**

FORGED

To forge means to shape by heating and hammering. We're going to heat up your body with metabolic-boosting plyometrics and then hammer it into shape with compound multi-muscle strength exercises.

Perform each set in order and rest 30 seconds after each set. Complete three rounds.

SET A

SQUAT JUMP	
0:30	**P**165

SINGLE-LEG PELVIC PEEL	
10x each side	**P**186

PISTOL SQUAT	
10x each side	**P**166

🕐 REST 0:30 before set B

SET B

BURPEE TO PULL-UP	
0:30	**P**178

ONE-ARM PUSH-UP	
5x each side	**P**197

PLYOMETRIC INVERTED ROW	
10x	**P**180

🕐 REST 0:30 before set C

SET C

PEDAL	
0:30	**P**182

T-STAND JUMP	
10x each side	**P**190

SQUAT TO L-SIT	
10x	**P**200

🕐 REST 0:30 before set D

ARMOUR ABS

Complete exercises in order and rest two minutes. Perform three rounds.

SET D

BURPEE TO CHIN-UP	
0:30	**P**192

PLYOMETRIC PUSH-UP	
10x	**P**136

ONE-ARM INVERTED ROW	
10x each side	**P**169

🕐 REST 0:30 before set E

SET E

SKIN THE CAT	
3x with a 10-second hold	**P**198

🕐 REST 0:30

🔄 REPEAT sets A–E for a total of three rounds

PIKE	
0:30	**P**053

HANGING LEG RAISE	
0:30	**P**110

HOLLOW BODY ROCKER	
0:30	**P**164

KNEE TUCK EXTENSIONS	
0:30	**P**188

DRAGON FLAG	
0:30	**P**196

HANGING REVERSE CURL	
0:30	**P**116

PLANCHE	
0:30	**P**167

🕐 REST 2:00

🔄 REPEAT Armour Abs for a total of three rounds

INFERNO

It's time to set your body ablaze with some high-intensity interval training and dynamic combination exercises such as Burpee to pull-ups. Adding speed not only increases the calorie-burning benefits of the workout but also adds instability. As your body compensates for the forces you create, it has to constantly adjust and counter the effects of gravity and motion. This will improve coordination and performance and help prevent injury.

When you're up against the clock, it's easy to lose track of the quality of your reps and instead focus only on quantity. Correct form should always be your first priority, so review the exercises thoroughly before you perform them at speed.

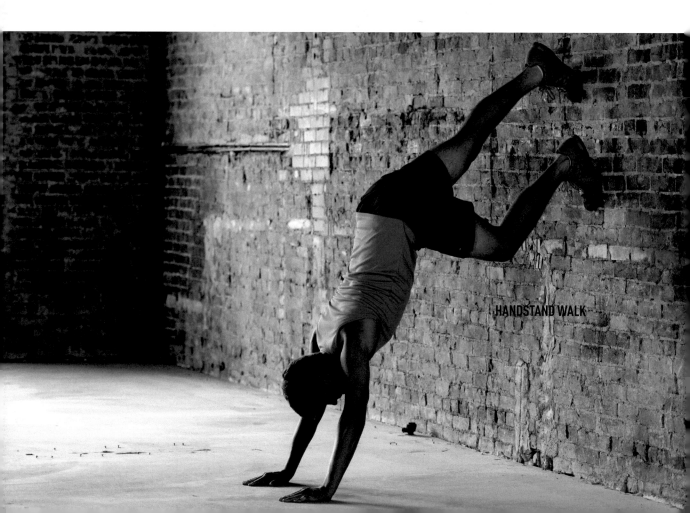

HANDSTAND WALK

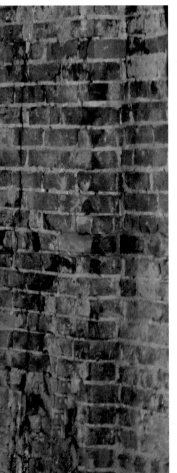

Perform all exercises in each set four times. Rest one minute between each set. Total time for the workout should be 27 minutes.

 SET A

BURPEE TO PULL-UP

| work 0:20, rest 0:10 | **P**178 |

SQUAT JUMP

| work 0:20, rest 0:10 | **P**165 |

ONE-ARM INVERTED ROW – RIGHT

| work 0:20, rest 0:10 | **P**169 |

ONE-ARM INVERTED ROW – LEFT

| work 0:20, rest 0:10 | **P**169 |

↻ REPEAT set A for a total of four rounds
🕐 REST 1:00 before set B

 SET B

BURPEE TO CHIN-UP

| work 0:20, rest 0:10 | **P**192 |

PEDAL

| work 0:20, rest 0:10 | **P**182 |

HANDSTAND WALK

| work 0:20, rest 0:10 | **P**162 |

HOLLOW BODY ROCKER

| work 0:20, rest 0:10 | **P**164 |

↻ REPEAT set B for a total of four rounds
🕐 REST 1:00 before set C

 SET C

TUCK JUMP BURPEE

| work 0:20, rest 0:10 | **P**194 |

T-STAND JUMP – RIGHT

| work 0:20, rest 0:10 | **P**190 |

T-STAND JUMP – LEFT

| work 0:20, rest 0:10 | **P**190 |

PLANCHE

| work 0:20, rest 0:10 | **P**167 |

↻ REPEAT set C for a total of four rounds
🕐 REST 1:00

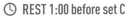
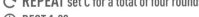

EVOLUTION

Fusing exercises from all three levels of this book, Evolution shows you just how far you've come in your bodyweight revolution. This workout evolves each set to take you from the base motion in Level 1 to the dynamic variation in Level 3.

> If three rounds of this workout is too challenging for you, perform only two, or adjust the reps on rounds two and three so you're working at 80 per cent of your max reps.

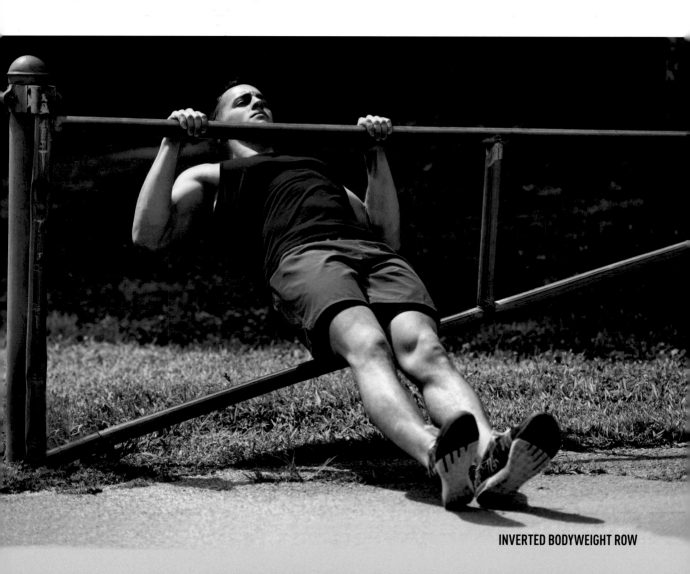

INVERTED BODYWEIGHT ROW

Perform each set in order with no rest between exercises. Rest one minute after each set. Complete three rounds.

SQUAT

10x	P081

STANDARD PRESS-UP

10x	P048

PULL-UP

10x	P056

ELBOW BRIDGE

0:30	P064

PELVIC PEEL

10x	P066

🕐 REST 1:00 before set B

SET B

SHRIMP SQUAT

10x each side	P118

STOP-AND-GO PRESS-UP

10x	P138

ARCHER PULL-UP

10x	P108

INVERTED BODYWEIGHT ROW

10x	P054

BUTTERFLY PEEL AND PIGEON PEEL

10x each	P122

🕐 REST 1:00 before set C

PISTOL SQUAT

10x each side	P166

PANCAKE PRESS-UP

10x	P176

BURPEE TO PULL-UP

10x	P178

ONE-ARM INVERTED ROW

0:10 each side	P169

SINGLE-LEG PELVIC PEEL

10x each side	P186

🕐 REST 1:00

↻ **REPEAT sets A–C for a total of three rounds**

ABDOMINATION
Complete six rounds. Total time: nine minutes.

HOLLOW BODY ROCKER

0:20	P164

FLUTTER UP

0:20	P177

DRAGON FLAG

0:20	P196

🕐 REST 0:30

↻ REPEAT Abdomination for a total of six rounds

SUPER CIRCUIT
THE BODYWEIGHT
500

This gruelling total body workout will demand 500 total reps of exercises from all levels. It will push you both mentally and physically. In exchange, you'll get increased endurance and improved athletic performance, and you'll shred fat. You have what it takes, but it will take all you've got!

Don't substitute any exercises or reduce the reps. Instead, when necessary, use the less difficult modification for each exercise to make the workout easier.

Complete all exercises in order and try to minimize rest time between exercises.

Exercise	Reps	Page
SQUAT	50x	P081
STANDARD PRESS-UP	50x	P048
SQUAT JUMP	25x	P165
PELVIC PEEL	25x	P066
PIKE	50x	P053
ALTERNATING LATERAL LUNGE	50x	P046
PULL-UP	25x	P056
BACK LUNGE	25x each leg	P075
MILITARY PRESS-UP	50x	P062
INVERTED BODYWEIGHT ROW	50x	P054
SKATER JUMP	50x	P130
BURPEE TO CHIN-UP	25x	P192

SUPER CIRCUIT
BEAST MODE

Beast Mode combines three of the toughest muscle-building sets from the workouts named after warriors and gods and breaks them up with metabolic "finishers" to create an epic Super Circuit. Beast Mode – ON!

Complete all sets and their exercises in order. Perform sets A, C, and E in pyramid format (decreasing reps per round where shown), and sets B and D as fast as possible. Rest 30 seconds between each set.

PISTOL SQUAT

10x each leg	P166

PANCAKE PRESS-UP

5x, 4x, 3x, 2x, 1x	P176

BURPEE TO PULL-UP

5x, 4x, 3x, 2x, 1x	P178

↻ REPEAT set A for five rounds in pyramid format
🕐 REST 0:30 before set B

1–2 PUSH

10x	P126

SKATER JUMP

20x	P130

SINGLE-LEG BURPEE

30x	P134

MOUNTAIN CLIMBER

40x	P043

↻ REPEAT set B for two rounds as fast as possible
🕐 REST 0:30 before set C

BULGARIAN SPLIT SQUAT

10x each leg	P124

SPIDERMAN PRESS-UP

5x, 4x, 3x, 2x, 1x	P103

ARCHER PULL-UP

5x, 4x, 3x, 2x, 1x	P108

↻ REPEAT set C for five rounds in pyramid format
🕐 REST 0:30 before set D

STANDARD PRESS-UP

10x	P048

X-JACK

20x	P072

BURPEE

30x	P060

MOUNTAIN CLIMBER

40x	P043

↻ REPEAT set D for two rounds as fast as possible
🕐 REST 0:30 before set E

SQUAT

10x	P081

STANDARD PRESS-UP

5x, 4x, 3x, 2x, 1x	P048

PULL-UP

5x, 4x, 3x, 2x, 1x	P056

↻ REPEAT set E for five rounds in pyramid format
🕐 REST 0:30
↻ REPEAT Beast Mode once more from set E to set A for the ultimate challenge (optional)

REDLINE

"Train 'til you redline" has become the unofficial tagline for my motorsport clients. The drivers I work with have to be strong and lean, and need incredible core strength. To achieve this goal, we fuse bodyweight resistance exercises and high-intensity interval training.

[If you struggle to recover between sets, extend the rest period to one minute.]

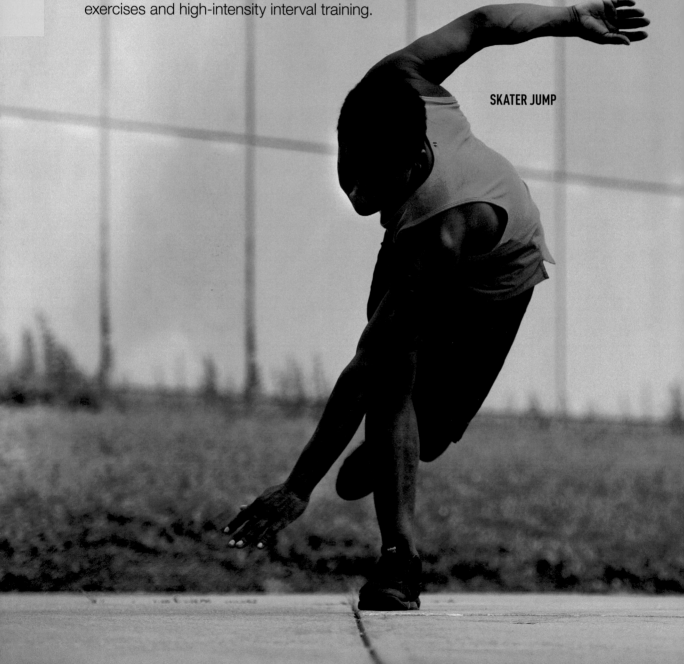

SKATER JUMP

Perform the exercises in each set in order. Rest 30 seconds between each set. Complete five rounds.

SET A

X-JACK

| 0:30 | **P**072 |

TUCK JUMP BURPEE

| 0:30 | **P**194 |

MOUNTAIN CLIMBER

| 0:30 | **P**043 |

BACKWARDS BURPEE

| 0:30 | **P**070 |

🕐 REST 0:30 before set B

SET B

PRESS-UP JACK

| 0:30 | **P**076 |

SKATER JUMP

| 0:30 | **P**130 |

1–2 PUSH

| 0:30 | **P**126 |

BURPEE TO CHIN-UP

| 0:30 | **P**192 |

🕐 REST 0:30

↻ **REPEAT sets A–B for a total of five rounds**

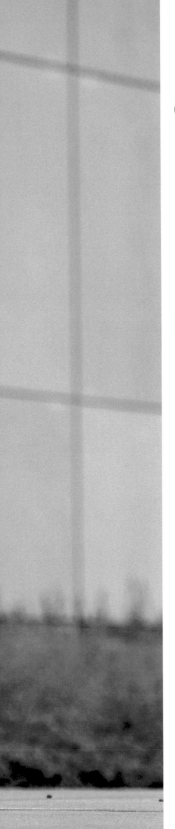

PROGRAMME

Each programme has six days of work and one day of rest. It's best to perform the workouts Monday to Saturday and rest on Sunday, but you can take a midweek rest day as needed. Don't switch the workouts within a programme, as this may have an adverse affect on rest time for a specific muscle group.

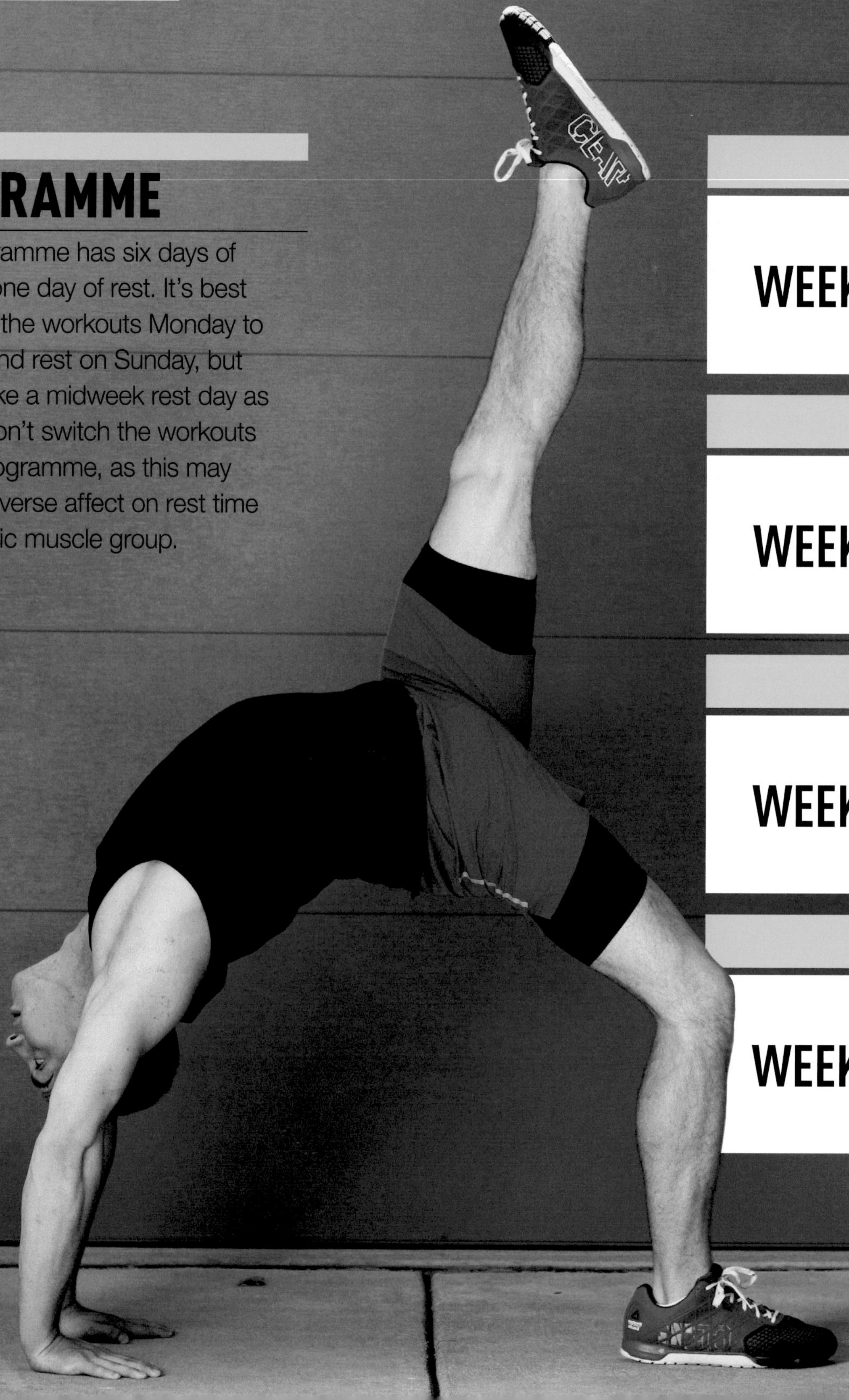

WEEK 1

WEEK 2

WEEK 3

WEEK 4

DAY **01**	DAY **02**	DAY **03**	DAY **04**	DAY **05**	DAY **06**
• ALEXANDER WORKOUT • FINISHER	• FOUNDATION • ARMOUR ABS	• SPARTACUS WORKOUT • TABATA-STYLE FINISHER	• PUSH/PULL POWER • ARMOUR ABS	• VLAD WORKOUT • FINISHER	• SUPER CIRCUIT THE BODYWEIGHT 500

DAY **08**	DAY **09**	DAY **10**	DAY **11**	DAY **12**	DAY **13**
• LEG HELL	• EVOLUTION • ABDOMINATION	• INFERNO	• FORGED • ARMOUR ABS	• REDLINE	• SUPER CIRCUIT BEAST MODE

DAY **15**	DAY **16**	DAY **17**	DAY **18**	DAY **19**	DAY **20**
• ALEXANDER WORKOUT • FINISHER	• FOUNDATION • ARMOUR ABS	• SPARTACUS WORKOUT • TABATA-STYLE FINISHER	• PUSH/PULL POWER • ARMOUR ABS	• VLAD WORKOUT • FINISHER	• SUPER CIRCUIT THE BODYWEIGHT 500

DAY **22**	DAY **23**	DAY **24**	DAY **25**	DAY **26**	DAY **27**
• LEG HELL	• EVOLUTION • ABDOMINATION	• INFERNO	• FORGED • ARMOUR ABS	• REDLINE	• SUPER CIRCUIT BEAST MODE

INDEX

ABOUT THE AUTHOR

Sean Bartram trains numerous professional athletes and celebrities, and is the official trainer to the Indianapolis Colts Cheerleaders. He has been featured by Shape, Popsugar, The Huffington Post, Fox, CBS, and Reuters. Bartram owns Core Pilates and Fitness in Carmel, Indiana, and is the author of High Intensity Interval Training for Women and Idiot's Guides: High Intensity Interval Training.

ACKNOWLEDGEMENTS

Thank you to everyone at DK for this opportunity, and to the incredibly talented group of people who have worked tirelessly behind the scenes to make this book a reality. An extra and very sincere thank you to Nathalie Mornu for her guidance and expertise as my editor, and special gratitude to Brook Farling for his unwavering support of me as an author.

Many thanks to the "Dream Team" of Matt Bowen and Nigel Wright. Your artistry behind the lens and your design excellence brings the text and exercises in this book to life.

Canterbury US (www.canterburyus.com) provided the entire wardrobe for this project and, having put their training apparel through its paces at the highest level myself, I can steadfastly recommend it to anyone picking up this book. A huge thank you to Canterbury US for their support of this project.

I can't give enough thanks to the outstanding athletes who grace each page of this book: Austin Bridenthal, Ray Boyden, Clayton Ford, and Blaize Monks, as well as fellow Brit and European champion Mark Freeman. An extra-special thank you to Mark. I'm looking forward to working and collaborating with him on many future projects. I strongly recommend checking out his website at www.freemantechnique.com.

Earnest thanks to each and every one of my clients, as each of you motivates and inspires me daily with your incredible drive and determination to meet your goals, not to mention the laughter and kindness you have all shared with me.

I would also like to thank the talented group of people and companies who represent or partner with me: Robbie, Wendy, and the team at Canterbury US; James and Blanca at SOS Rehydrate; and Jeff and Alex of Frog Performance.

Thank you to Jack Harvey, Jack Hawksworth, Kelly Tilley, Erin Bell, Ashli Pickens, Mary Worline, Dwayne Allen, Matt Overton, and the incredible ladies of Colts Cheer who demand nothing but the best from me and help me find it with their toughness, dedication, and "all in, all the time" mentality.

For my parents: thank you for the greatest gift a parent can offer – belief. I don't say it often enough: I love and miss you.

Finally, a heartfelt thank you to Rochelle and Chloe. I'm proud of you – each of you – for your own wonderfully unique gifts. You make me laugh, keep me humble, and put up with me even when I have expended all my physical or mental energy. You always find a way to show me your love when I need it the most.